AGING, DISABILITY AND INDEPENDENCE

Assistive Technology Research Series

The Assistive Technology Research Series (ATR) aims to disseminate and archive assistive technology research summaries widely through publishing proceedings, monographs, and edited collective works. The series aspires to become the primary world-wide source of information in assistive technology research, through publishing state-of-the-science material across all continents. ATR defines assistive technology (AT) as any tool, equipment, system, or service designed to help develop, maintain or improve a person with a disability to function in all aspects of his or her life. Assistive technology helps people of all ages who may have a broad range of disabilities or limitations. The ATR series will accept manuscripts and proposals for a wide range of relevant topics.

Volume 22

Recently published in this series

Vol. 21. A. Mihailidis, J. Boger, H. Kautz and L. Normie (Eds.), Technology and Aging – Selected Papers from the 2007 International Conference on Technology and Aging

Vol. 20. G. Eizmendi, J.M. Azkoitia and G. Craddock (Eds.), Challenges for Assistive Technology – AAATE 07

Vol. 19. C. Nugent and J.C. Augusto (Eds.), Smart Homes and Beyond – ICOST2006, 4th International Conference On Smart homes and health Telematics

Vol. 18. W.C. Mann and A. Helal (Eds.), Promoting Independence for Older Persons with Disabilities – Selected Papers from the 2006 International Conference on Aging, Disability and Independence

Vol. 17. H. Mollenkopf, F. Marcellini, I. Ruoppila, Z. Széman and M. Tacken (Eds.), Enhancing Mobility in Later Life – Personal Coping, Environmental Resources and Technical Support. The Out-of-Home Mobility of Older Adults in Urban and Rural Regions of Five European Countries

Vol. 16. A. Pruski and H. Knops (Eds.), Assistive Technology: From Virtuality to Reality – AAATE 2005

ISSN 1383-813X

Aging, Disability and Independence

Selected Papers from the 4th International Conference on Aging, Disability and Independence (2008)

Edited by

William C. Mann

College of Public Health and Health Professions, University of Florida, Gainesville, FL USA

IOS Press

Amsterdam • Berlin • Oxford • Tokyo • Washington, DC

Previously published by the University of Florida, Gainesville, FL, USA.

ISBN 978-1-58603-902-8
Library of Congress Control Number: 2008936295

Publisher
IOS Press
Nieuwe Hemweg 6B
1013 BG Amsterdam
Netherlands
fax: +31 20 687 0019
e-mail: order@iospress.nl

Distributor in the UK and Ireland
Gazelle Books Services Ltd.
White Cross Mills
Hightown
Lancaster LA1 4XS
United Kingdom
fax: +44 1524 63232
e-mail: sales@gazellebooks.co.uk

Distributor in the USA and Canada
IOS Press, Inc.
4502 Rachael Manor Drive
Fairfax, VA 22032
USA
fax: +1 703 323 3668
e-mail: iosbooks@iospress.com

PRINTED IN THE NETHERLANDS

Aging, Disability and Independence
W.C. Mann (Ed.)
IOS Press, 2008

Preface

This book includes 15 full-length papers submitted for the Fourth International Conference on Aging, Disability, and Independence (ICADI) and held in St. Petersburg, Florida, USA from February 20-23, 2008. These papers reflect five ICADI tracks: Livable Homes and Communities, Smart Homes and Robotics, Transportation, Work, and Assistive Technology and one ICADI theme: Consumer Perspective.

The broad objectives of ICADI are the synthesis and translation of knowledge about disability and aging, and approaches to maintaining independence and quality of life, while fostering collaborations to support future research in this area. ICADI promotes knowledge translation through a mix of invited and submitted presentations, poster sessions, and networking opportunities with experts from around the world. ICADI-2008, as with previous ICADI's, has provided investigators the opportunity to present their research and development work at the Conference, and to have that work receive wider dissemination through this book, and through the ICADI Conference Proceedings, available at www.icadi.phhp.ufl.edu.

The First International Conference on Aging, Disability and Independence (ICADI) was held in December 1999, in Washington, D.C, and was attended by nearly 300 participants. The Second ICADI was held in Washington in 2003 as the University of Florida Rehabilitation Engineering Research Center on Aging State of the Science Conference and then again in 2006 in St. Petersburg, Florida where over 525 people from 32 countries participated. ICADI is unique in bringing together researchers, practitioners, business leaders and people involved in research and development and related aging policy to focus on issues of aging, disability and independence.

The major focus of ICADI on aging and disability related services, research and development, and policy, brings together a rich mix of motivated and talented individuals (multi-disciplinary and engaged in different sectors and types of organizations) who ultimately impact these services. Further, as an international conference, ICADI provides the opportunity to learn more about the successes, challenges and different approaches to the independence-related needs of elders in different countries. Key Groups include: (1) Research and Development personnel; (2) Practitioners / Service Providers; (3) Policymakers; (4) Business Representatives; (5) Consumers; (6) Professional and Graduate Students.

ICADI 2008 has the support of almost 100 major organizations in "spreading the word" on the conference. We thank them for their help with ICADI. Further, we have a number of organizations, companies and agencies that provide financial support for ICADI, each supporting a specific ICADI track, special event, or need. Without their support, ICADI would not be possible, and we thank each of them. The National Institute on Disability and Rehabilitation Research (NIDRR) is the lead sponsor for this book. We offer a special thank you to NIDRR, for this book, and their past support of the Rehabilitation Engineering Research Center on Aging.

William C. Mann
Distinguished Professor and ICADI Conference Chair
University of Florida

Contents

Aging, Disability and Independence
W.C. Mann (Ed.)
IOS Press, 2008

doi:10.3233/978-1-58603-902-8-1

Housing in Response to the Human Life Cycle

Emory Baldwin[1]
[1] ZAI inc, 5228 Kirkwood Pl. N., Seattle, WA 98103, USA

Abstrast: The essence of Universal Design principles rests in the fundamental premise of a flexible, supportive, and nondiscriminatory environment. Unfortunately, conventional housing is generally designed for the singular needs of a romanticized nuclear family without the allowance for disabilities, transitions or creative living solutions. The average household composition is becoming increasingly varied as our society becomes more diverse. The traditional household makeup has expanded to include elderly relatives, caregivers, unrelated adults, and even home businesses. The rapidly aging population and longer life expectancies are leading to a greater number of people with physical and cognitive disabilities. Additionally, housing prices are high for first-time buyers, while many 'empty nesters' have more space than they need. These trends demand a new approach to designing environments, which would better accommodate people's changing situations and their varying abilities. By designing flexibility into homes from the beginning, it is possible to reduce one's frequent need to move and also to enable our elders to age in place. With a home's layout and structure designed to allow for a number of varied floor plans, it may be easily modified when the need arises, thus reducing potential remodeling costs and waste, increasing the marketability of a home, and contributing to more stable and sustainable communities. With this truly universal approach, a home would be more than just a shelter. It would be a person's most valuable tool, supporting them throughout their lifespan.

Keywords: Flexible Housing; Lifespan Design; Trans-generational; Sustainable; Affordable

Introduction

The average household in the United States has changed dramatically over the last fifty years, and it is impossible to predict how it will change over the next fifty. As the compositions of households become increasingly varied, and society becomes more diverse, it is appropriate to re-think the notion of the traditional family and the buildings in which they live. The traditional household structure has expanded to include elderly relatives, caregivers and unrelated adults. Today's multi-cultural and multi-generational households require buildings that are responsive, flexible, and transformable as opposed to fixed, rigid, and unchangeable.

"In a society where the most common type of household is led by those who live alone and where the scattered family is almost a cultural institution, many grandparents, adult children and grandchildren are gathering to live under the same roof. The last (U.S.) census showed these 'multi-generational households' – defined as those of three or more generations – growing faster than any other type of housing arrangement. The number of multigenerational households is still relatively small: 4.2 million, or 4 percent of all types. However, they grew by 38 percent from 1990 to 2000, and professionals in real estate and the building industry say the trend has accelerated since then [4]."

The makeup of American society is changing as the number of disabled and elderly people rapidly increases. The baby-boomer population is aging, and medical technology is assisting people with disabilities to survive into older age. According to the U.S. Census Bureau, the population of Americans aged 65 and over is projected to double by 2030, while those aged 85 and over is expected to almost triple[1].

The physiological life cycle takes a person through different stages of development and growth and then eventually leads them to deterioration and fragility. Many elderly people are forced to enter an institution prematurely simply because their own homes are unable to accommodate the disabilities they develop. Design of a home must take into account the fact that the occupants' abilities will vary over their lifetime. Disabilities can come at any time, and the home must be able to accommodate them. Some disabilities are temporary such as sports injuries, while others are permanent. Regardless of the duration of the disability, a well-designed environment can improve the quality of life of the occupant.

More and more Americans are finding it difficult to pay for housing costs in today's economy. More middle-aged and older couples who already own homes often find themselves with substantial amounts of extra space after their children have left home. Conventional housing stock generally does not respond to this growing problem. How can a house itself enable affordability and assist in paying for some of its costs? How can a house respond to the needs of more space, and conversely make use of too much space? There is a need to design flexibility into the home so that the residents can vary the amount and the use of space according to their changing needs throughout their lives.

New Approach to Housing

Universal Design

Housing is too frequently designed for the "average" person with "average" physical ability when, in reality, few people meet this description of "average". People range greatly in size and physical and mental abilities, and they experience many changes throughout their lives. When designing a house, designers tend to respond to a "snapshot" of the client as he or she looks today, and they forget to allow for changes in the client's physical ability and lifestyle over time. Good design should accommodate all users, and when all users are taken into account equally from the beginning, rather than as an afterthought, the resulting design can be intelligent, sensitive, exciting, and non-exclusive.

"Universal design is the design of products and environments to be usable by all people, to the greatest extent possible, without the need for adaptation or specialized design [3]." While this is true on the micro level of ergonomics and accessibility, there are other issues involved with the macro level of society and people's changing spatial requirements which call for flexibility, so as to allow one's home to expand, contract and shift to the larger rhythms of life.

Lifespan Design

Lifespan Design goes beyond the traditional scope of universal design and embraces an even broader design methodology that addresses the full spectrum of the human life cycle. A person's needs change between different phases of his or her life cycle, and also between different living arrangements. (Figure 1) A married couple with children, for example, has different needs than a household of unrelated, sharing adults. The activities performed by a young couple with an infant are likely different than those performed by an elderly person with a caregiver. Housing should be able to respond to these lifestyle changes as well as the physical and cognitive changes described previously. When housing can support many choices and needs, it becomes a dynamic and transformative environment enabling one to "age-in-place" with dignity and empowerment.

Residential Flexibility

Although universal design strives to create environments that are more usable by the largest extent of the population as possible, it does not mean that there is always one idealized way of doing something that works best for everyone. Flexibility is necessary, not only for the natural evolution of living situations and household configurations that occur within a dwelling over time, but also for the unexpected occurrences that relate to changes in physical and cognitive abilities.

There are different levels of flexibility that should be represented in the design of lifespan housing. First, there are daily adjustments that may need to be made, such as raising or lowering a counter, sink, or toilet seat. These changes are usually

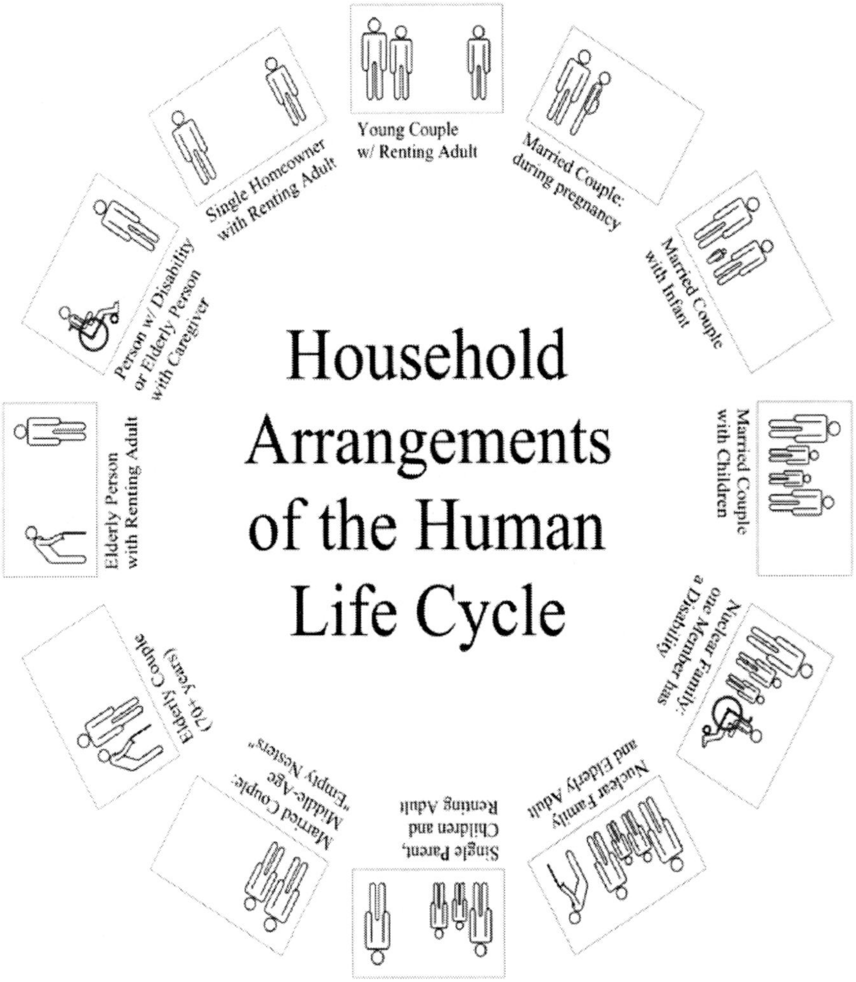

Figure 1. Household Arrangements of the Human Life Cycle

due to physical differences between the various occupants of the home. Secondly, there are adjustments that might be done from month-to-month or from year-to-year. Movable closets and shelving units can be easily rearranged to modify the layout of a room or an area of the home. These types of changes reflect subtle differences in occupants' preferences and spatial and privacy requirements. Adjustable height closet rods allow for the natural growth of a resident or for a change from one type of clothing to another. Lastly, there are the major alterations that occur such as relocation of walls, changes in room function and external additions. These infrequent transformations are due to radical changes in the lifestyle, physical and mental condition, or living arrangement of the occupants.

While the general aim is to make housing more flexible, there must be some features that are fixed, both for practicality and to give some ordering structure to the layout. For example, a fixed "core" in a home would include a vertical duct for mechanical services, a staircase, and an elevator shaft that could be used as valuable closet space until an elevator was needed. By fixing the location of features that pass between levels, future renovation would be simpler and less expensive.

Breaking the home down into different zones (one for permanent occupation and one for expansion) would allow the home to be more flexible and respond to the changing needs and living situations of the owners. The provision of an area that could serve as an accessory apartment or a caregiver's residence would aid occupants at different stages of the life cycle. It makes sense to generally locate activities and functions that will always be required in the permanent-occupation zone, and temporary functions in the expansion zone. This strategy will reduce the need to change the entire layout in the future.

By designing flexibility into homes from the beginning, it may be possible to reduce one's need to move to a new home and also to prevent, or at least postpone, an elderly occupant's move to an institution. Future flexibility can be allowed for by designing the building layout and structure to be equally accommodating of a number of varied floor plans so that the homes may be easily modified when the need arises. Building flexibility into dwellings is not only humane, but it "increases the practical value of housing for everyone, thus creating better rentability" and marketability [5].

Guidelines to Enable Flexibility

The following are important guidelines that should be incorporated into the design of a home, to make it flexible enough to support a person throughout his or her lifespan:

Location near Amenities:

The feasibility of a home designed for one's lifetime depends in large part upon the nearby location of a range of amenities that would provide services and opportunities for recreation. Such amenities would include medical clinics, pharmacies, grocery stores, activity centers, libraries, schools, parks and public transportation. The availability of in-home services, such as home delivery of groceries, house visits by health care workers, special transportation and house cleaning, maintenance and repair, would also be extremely helpful to elderly persons, people with disabilities, or people with busy careers. Access to friends, family and society is important as well.

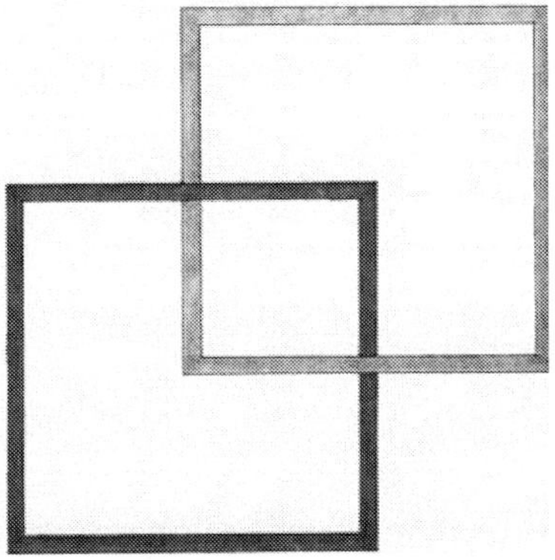

Figure 2: Distinction between Primary and Accessory Functions

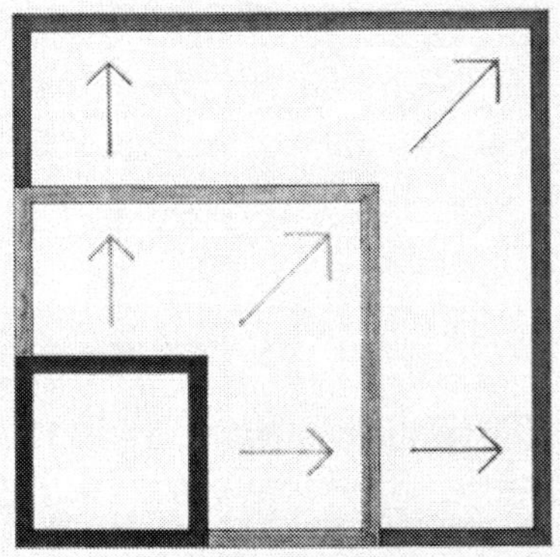

Figure 3: Varying Amounts of Accessory Space

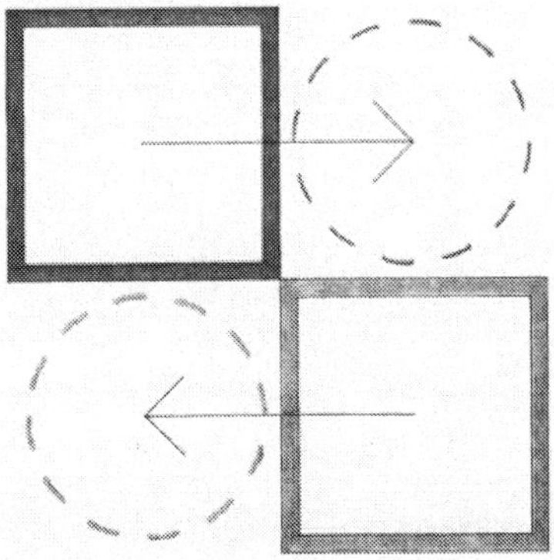

Figure 4: Private Outdoor Space

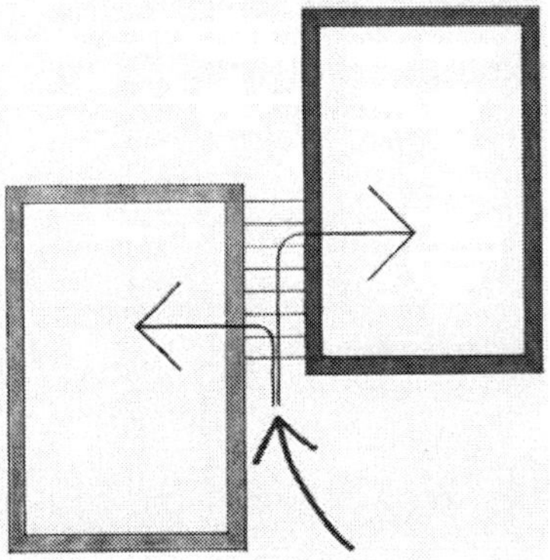

Figure 5: Private Entrance for Accessory Area

Distinction between Primary and Accessory Function (Figure 2):
Separate the core spaces from those that are only needed temporarily, so that accessory areas may be visually defined and differentiated from primary homeowner's realm. This separation also works to create privacy between primary and accessory areas.
Varying Amounts of Accessory Space (Figure 3):
The amount of space that a household requires changes over time. By allowing the dwelling to be divided in a number of ways, the primary occupant can rent out or rezone space as their needs evolve.
Private Outdoor Space (Figure 4):
The primary and accessory parts of the dwelling should each have their own private outdoor space. Such a space should provide privacy not only from the street and alley, but also from other parts of the building.
Private Entrance for Accessory Area (Figure 5):
Both work areas and accessory apartments should be accessible without entering the zone of the primary homeowner.
Central Vertical Circulation Core (Figure 6):
Both the stairway and the dedicated vertical shaft should be

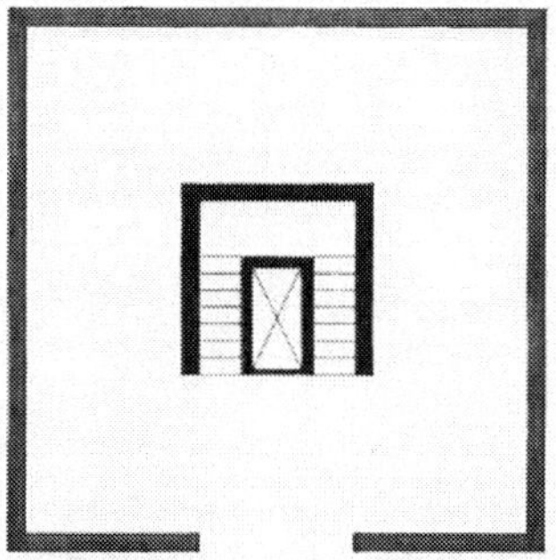

Figure 6: Central Vertical Circulation Core

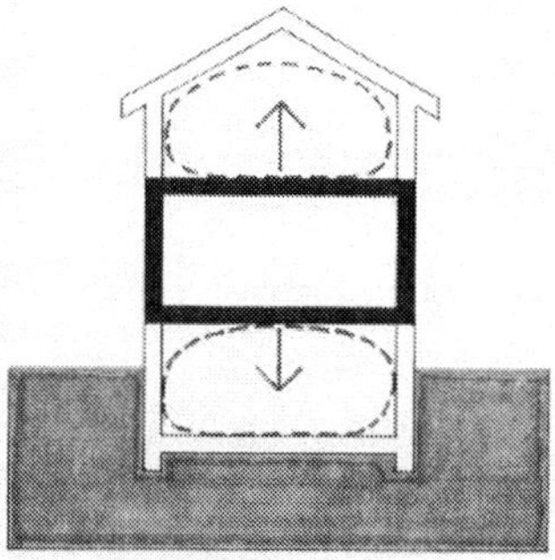

Figure 7: Areas for Future Expansion

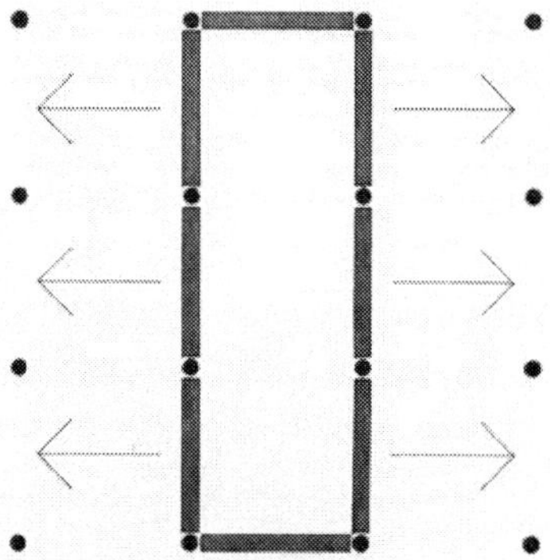

Figure 8: Flexible Layout

centrally located within the home, near the entrance. The two means of vertical circulation should be closely associated with each other so that one is not further away or more difficult to access than the other.

Areas for Future Expansion (Figure 7):

The inclusion of a sunroom, courtyard, attic or basement provides the option for future inward expansion. The incorporation of such unfinished spaces in the original design makes future additions less expensive and raises the value of the dwelling.

Flexible Layout (Figure 8):

Living arrangements and needs change over time. Allow the building to be flexible so that the layout may be easily changed, and so that an area can be used for different functions over time.

Minimization of Load Bearing Walls (Figure 9):

Use a post and beam, or structural panel system in order to maximize the level of flexibility of the building. Large areas of load-bearing wall inhibit the building's ability to change over time.

Zones of Building Services (Figure 10):

Relocating plumbing can be one of the most difficult parts of home renovation. Organize the plumbing and other services into logical zones to allow simpler future renovation. Create a network of plumbing "ducts" and "trenches" to which future wet areas may easily connect [3].

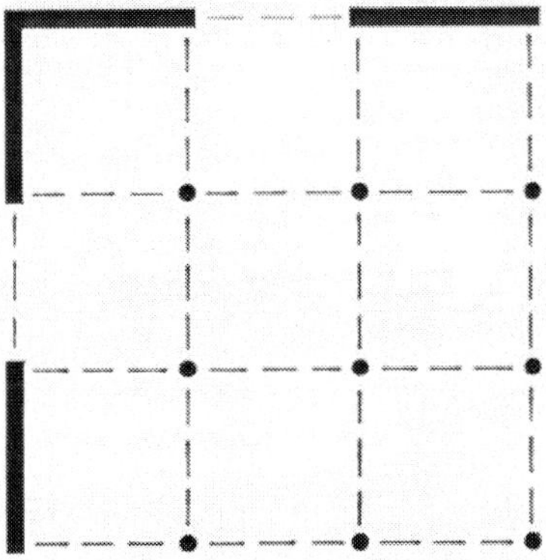

Figure 9: Minimization of Load Bearing Walls

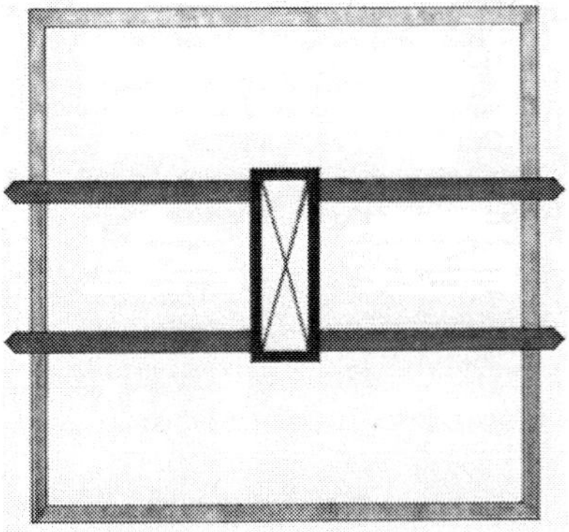

Figure 10: Zones of Building Services

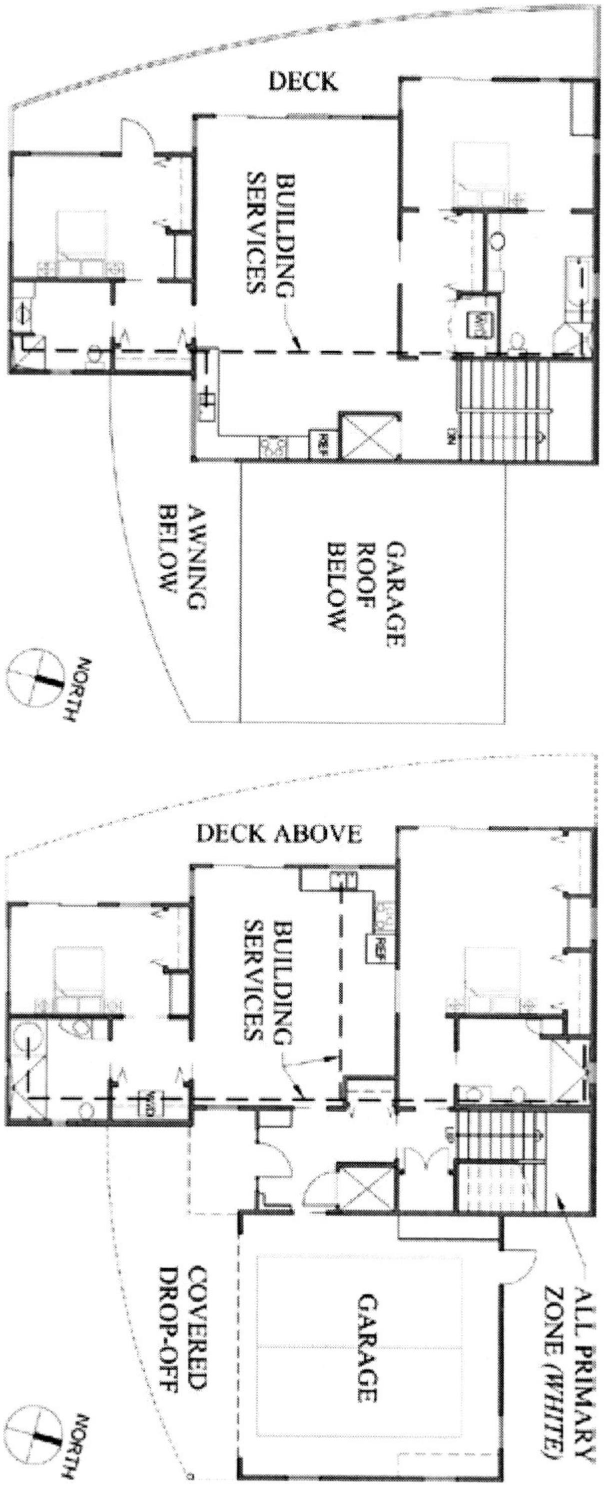

Figure 11: Universal Design Showroom - Variation 1: Single Family House

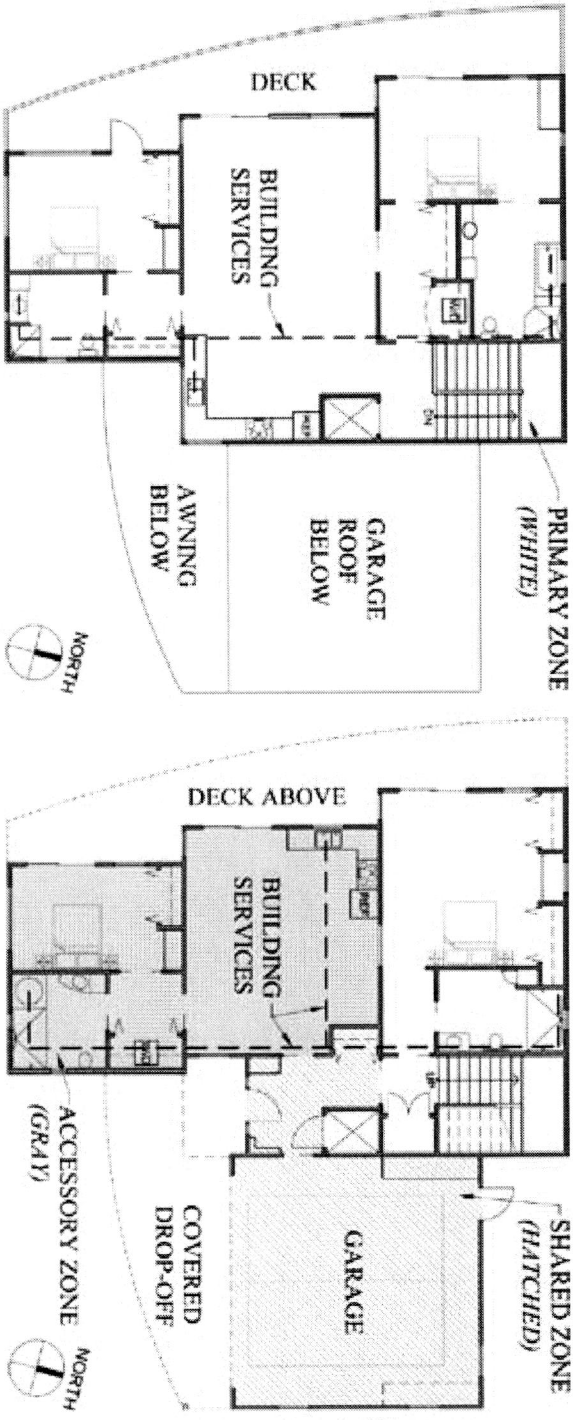

Figure 12 - Universal Design Showroom - Variation 2: Primary Home and Home Office / Rental

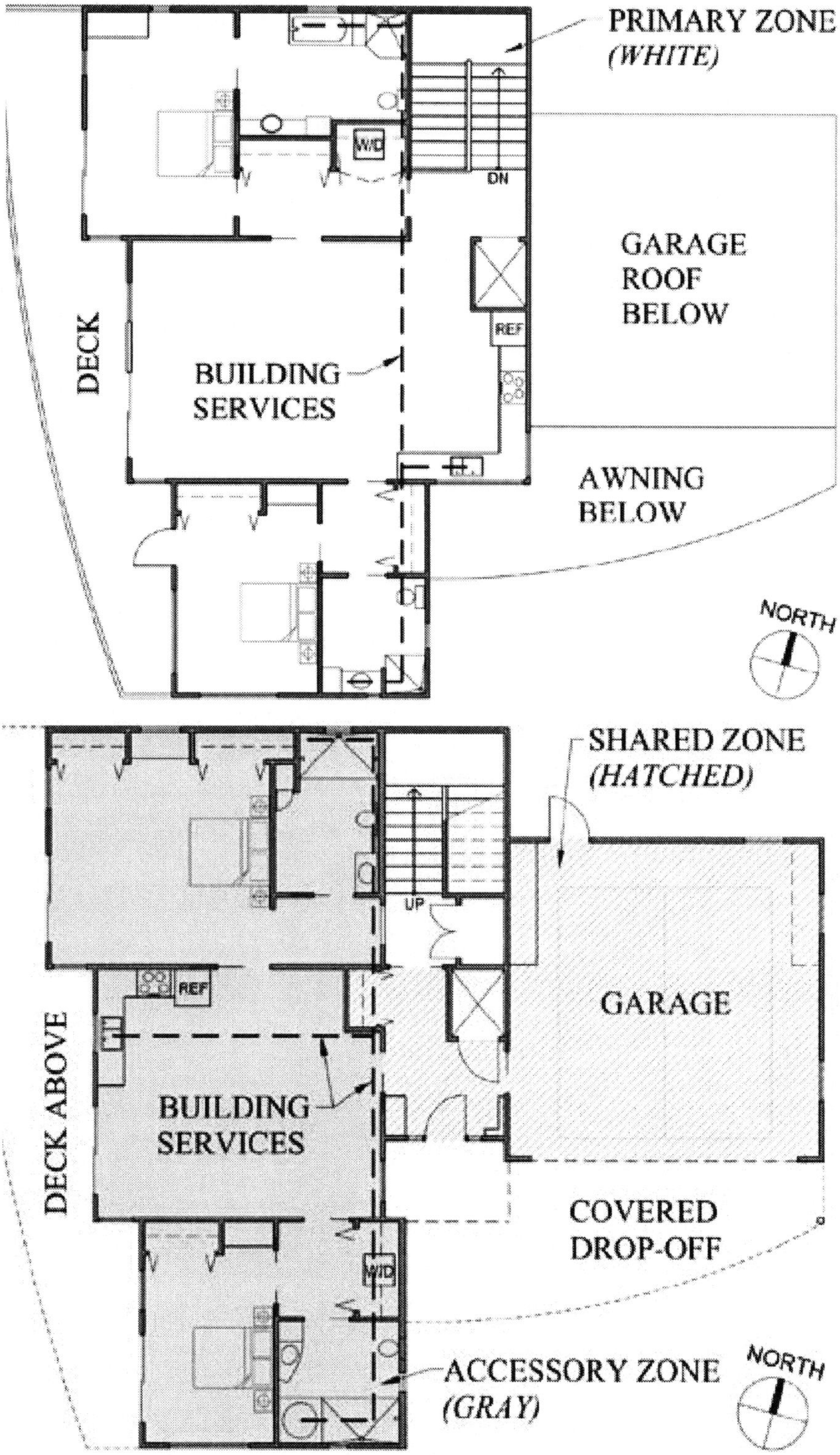

Figure 13 - Universal Design Showroom - Variation 3: Duplex

Examples

Universal Design Showroom / Duplex, Sitka, Alaska, USA

This project, currently being designed, is a good example of a flexible dwelling. Several layout possibilities have been designed into the structure from the beginning, thus providing a number of options for use. It can either be used as one large single family residence (Figure 11), a smaller home with a home office (Figure 12), a duplex with two equally sized units (Figure 13), or a medium-size home with a rental unit or caregiver unit. The initial use of the building will be a primary residence for the owner on the upper floor and a showroom (of universal design products and ideas) for the owner's business on the ground floor. The entire building will be universally designed, and each of the four bathrooms will showcase different universally designed layouts. One of the bedroom / office suites on the ground floor will be a multiple-use space that can function as a living room, family room or studio. Furthermore, by the use of movable walls, this suite can be manipulated to belong to either the upper unit or lower unit, as shown in the diagrams below. This flexibility of use will provide greater functionality and allow the building to respond to the owner's changing needs and living situations.

The owners, who run a home modification business, have been very involved in the design of the project, and have pushed for showing best practices of Universal Design. In addition, the owners have encouraged the incorporation of four different layouts for the bathrooms to best show a range of options for their clients' varying situations. Due to the cold climate of the site, the owners wished to incorporate an "arctic entry", which is essentially an airlock between doors. Not only does this reduce

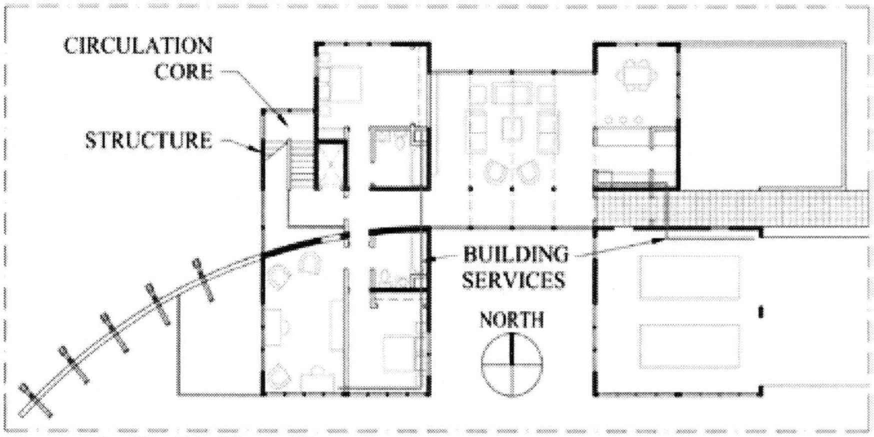

Figure 14 - Flexible House Upper Level

the amount of heat transmission between the inside and outside of the building, but it also separates the inner and outer doors of an entry, thus making them easier to manage. Additionally, large (4 foot) overhangs and pressure equalized "rain screen" cladding help to protect the structure from the heavy rainfall that southeast Alaska experiences. A covered drop-off area also protects people coming and going from the house, and keeps moisture away from the level entry.

Flexible House, Seattle, Washington, USA:

Another home was designed by the author in 1997 to transform according to its occupant's evolving spatial needs. The arrangement of the structure provides many options for dividing up the dwelling. The primary zone can be a self-contained, one-story unit when the primary occupant does not need much space. (Figure 14) One or both levels of the accessory area can be rented out, depending on how much space is required by the primary occupant. In the situation where the primary homeowner has a large household, the entire dwelling can become one large unit.

This single-family dwelling was positioned on its site to allow two levels of entry: a formal entry on the street side and a less formal entry on the alley side. A circulation spine runs through the middle of the house, defining the primary and accessory zones. The circulation corridor also acts as a noise barrier between the two zones. This allows privacy between parents'

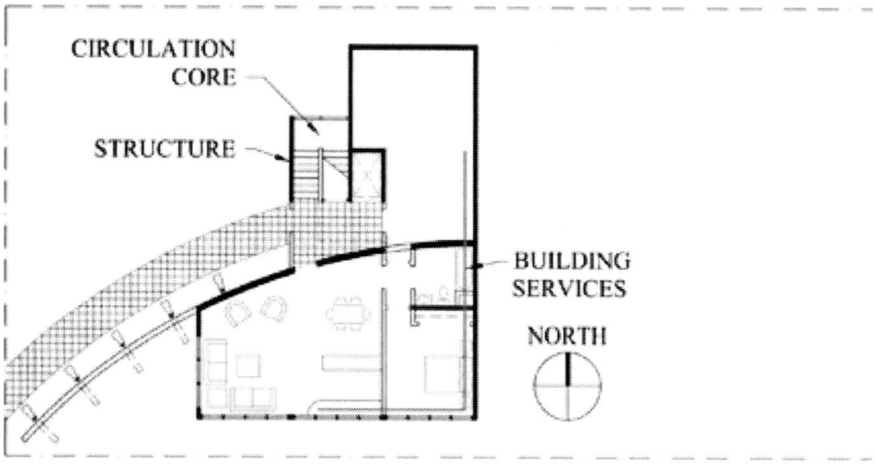

Figure 15 - Flexible House

and children's areas when the house is one unit, or between primary homeowner's and renter's areas when the house is divided. The vertical circulation core consists of both a stairway and a dedicated vertical space that can be used as closets until an elevator is needed (Figure 15).

The house is laid out on a twelve-and-a-half foot (375 cm) grid, so that there is always at least twelve feet (360 cm) between major points of structure. This creates a good dimension for most rooms and allows non-load-bearing internal walls to be placed where smaller spaces are needed. Plumbing, wiring and other building services are arranged in strategically placed ducts and trenches, which allow a range of locations for kitchens and baths, and simplify future renovation.

The layout of this house assumes universal design as a point of departure. The 12'-6" (375 cm) dimension of the dwelling's structural grid is designed to accommodate accessible spaces such as bathrooms, hallways and food preparation areas. For example, an 8' x 8' (240 cm x 240 cm) accessible bathroom, a 42" (105 cm) wide hallway and a 6" (15 cm) wall all fit within the 12' (360 cm) space between structural points. There are no steps or level changes within the dwelling aside from that of the vertical circulation core. This allows the whole house to be fully accessible, and prevents any area from being unusable by persons with disabilities.

Parkinson's Disease Supportive Living Facility, Mountlake Terrace, Washington, USA:

Another project currently in the design stage, is an assisted living facility that is exclusively for people living with Parkinson's disease. The project will be much smaller than a typical assisted living facility, and the aim is to make it appear and feel like a series of small houses, rather than a large institutional facility. Since it will be small, yet need the same common spaces as a larger project, the spaces will have to be very efficient in size, and many of them will have to serve multiple functions. Common spaces will be able to open up for large gatherings, or close off for smaller groups, thus allowing a number of simultaneous activities to occur. (Figure 16) Bedrooms will be laid out so that they can function for a variety of users. Both long-term residents and short-term respite guests must be accommodated, yet the proportions of each will likely continually change. Occasionally,

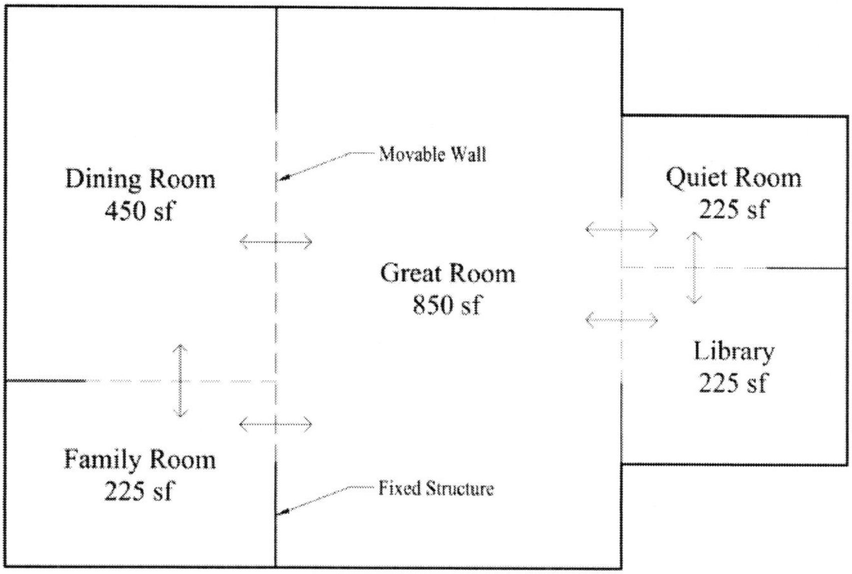

Figure 16 - Parkinson's Disease Facility: Example of Flexible Multi-purpose Spaces

family members will also need to sleep overnight. Designing the bedrooms to be flexible will enable the facility to respond to the changing mix of users and also help to reduce vacancy. Since the owners perceive a growing demand for such a facility, the building will be designed for future growth. Future expansion of the building needs to be easily accommodated by the preliminary layout of the structure (Figure 17).

Conclusion

The concepts of both Universal Design and Lifespan Design are applicable to the full array of dwelling types, as well as other building types, since all people and organizations experience changes throughout their life cycles. Single-family homes, townhouses, apartment buildings, and even commercial and institutional buildings each have ways that they can be made to adapt to the changing needs of their respective users. The principles of both universal design and flexibility of layout would allow homes of any category to better support their occupants over a lifespan, and reduce their need to move. It could be argued that apartment buildings would have less turn over (and thus lower vacancy) if the apartments could respond to the residents' evolving needs.

This same idea would contribute to stronger and more stable

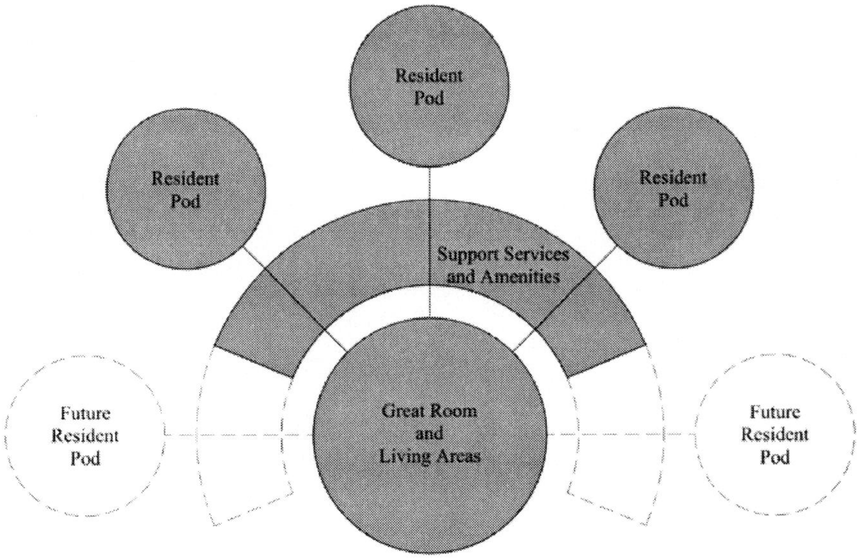

Figure 17 - Parkinson's Disease Facility: Overall Conceptual Layout

neighborhoods, since people would have less reason to move, be able to stay in place for longer, and get to know their neighbors better. This concept would not only help to sustain enduring communities, but it would also provide an environmentally sustainable alternative to wasteful remodeling. Furthermore, homes that are both universally designed and designed for a lifespan would allow many affordable options for people to retain their homes when their needs change and they need more or less space.

The realm of Universal Design should be expanded to accommodate people's changing social and economic situations in addition to their varying physical abilities. It should engage all aspects of sensible, quality design, including global issues of sustainability, affordability, and human dignity.

With this approach, a home can be more than just a shelter, its potential is to be a person's most valuable tool and asset, supporting them throughout their lifespan, and thus it is fundamentally sustainable, affordable, inclusive and truly UNIVERSAL.

References

[1] Gunts, Edward, 1994. "Housing the Elderly", Architecture, October, vol. 83, no. 10, p.83.

[2] Kendall, Stephen, 1993. "Open Building for Housing", Progressive Architecture, vol 74, no. 11, p. 95.

[3] Mace, Ron, Available at: http://www.design.ncsu.edu/cud/about_ud/aboutud.htm

[4] Navarro, Mireya, 2006. "Families Add 3rd Generation to Households". New York Times, May 25.

[5] van der Voordt, Theo J. M., 1990. "Building Adaptable Housing – From Theory to Practice", Architecture & Behavior, vol. 6, no. 1, p. 19.

Aging, Disability and Independence
W.C. Mann (Ed.)
IOS Press, 2008

doi:10.3233/978-1-58603-902-8-19

Housing for an Ageing Society: Adapting Housing Design toward Universality is the Minimum Requirement for Inclusion

Satoshi Kose[1]
[1]Shizuoka University of Art and Culture,
Hamamatsu, 430-8533 Japan

Abstract: The world is ageing, and Japan is no exception. Japan is the fastest graying society in the world, and a quarter of its population will be over age 65 by 2014. It is inevitable that many older people will experience difficulties in the environment due to capability deterioration. To address these environmental problems, the Japanese Construction Ministry inititated in 1987 a five-year research and development project on design for the ageing society. Design for All Ages was set as the key concept, discarding the traditional idea of "special design for the aged." It is a clear departure from age segregation that occurs with sheltered housing. Design for All Ages assumes that residents will age in place, and that the dwellings will be able to respond to the changing needs of residents. After all, dwellings are an important component of a person's life, and disability (particularly age-related disability) should not adversely affect people.

During the research and development stages of Design for All ages, we integrated existing knowledge with new ideas derived from experiments. Basic concepts for dwellings that have been adopted include: Safety; accessibility; usability; and affordability. These concepts can be interpreted in terms of design guidelines:

1) Basically flat floor. No door sills, no step differences, unless vitally necessary.
2) Handrail installation at critical places such as stairs, bathroom, toilet, and entrances.
3) Wider corridors and doors.

The final Guidelines were based on the discussions of effectiveness, design and economic feasibility, climatic conditions, and cultural tradition. However, simply issuing guidelines does not ensure they will be put into practice. Japan has a strong mechanism for implementation: the Japan Housing Loan Corporation (HLC). The HLC has given prospective clients lower interest rates for housing mortgages, and has been a driving force of economic growth since its establishment in 1950. The Corporation took a decisive step in 1996 in establishing barrier-free or energy conscious design to be eligible for lowest interest rates. Along with the Guidelines, consumer education was provided through various approaches. As a result, construction of barrier-free dwellings increased, and the majority of newer dwellings were built to be basically barrier-free.

Older dwellings were and still are poor in terms of barrier-free design. In addition, aged persons who are more vulnerable and experiencing difficulties in daily living tend to live in problematic dwellings with many barriers. To address these problems, the Japan Housing Finance Agency (the successor to HLC) assists with remodelling of older people's dwelling, though most government subsidized mortgages have been discontinued.

Keywords: Design for ageing, dwellings, housing policy, and universal design.

Introduction

Japan has become one of the oldest societies in the world. It is estimated that more than a quarter of the population in Japan will be over age 65 by 2015. Care of older persons by their family members is becoming more difficult. Minimum barrier-free physical environments will be needed to avoid inconveniences during daily living. To solve these problems, the Ministry of Construction initiated a five-year research and development project on design for the aged society in 1987. The author took the leading role in defining the aim of the project, and put "design for all ages" as the key concept, discarding the traditional idea of special design for the aged. In Japan in June 1994, the "Act on Accessible and Usable Buildings for the Aged and Physically Disabled Persons" was passed, and in June 1995, "Design Guidelines of Dwellings for the Ageing Society" was issued. This legislation and the Design Guidelines are similar to ADA and FHAA Guidelines in the United States. The goal of this Japanese law and Guidelines is to enhance opportunities for older people to live, go out and move around in the community. It is a clear departure from age segregation that occurs with sheltered housing. It assumes that residents will age in place, and that the dwellings will be able to respond to the residents' changing needs. Comparison of housing policies for the older persons in different countries (including Japan) can be found in Brink[1].

Design for all Ages: Universal Design Concept

During the development stages of Design for All Ages, the author integrated existing knowledge with new ideas derived from experiments. Results of these experiments are reported elsewhere [3, 4, 5, 14, 15,17]. The basic concepts for dwellings that were adopted include:

1) The dwellings should be livable 30 years after they are built.
2) Safety, comfort, and usability must be ensured for all residents.
3) Required level should not be too high to be universal.
4) Dwellings should be adaptable to meet new requirements in response to changing needs.
5) Design and facilities should be given choice depending on the needs of the residents.

To translate these concepts into practice, the following areas had to be addressed:

1) Safety of the residents (no tripping risk on floors, etc.).
2) Physical support for negotiation (such as handrails).
3) Potential for single floor living (as opposed to stair use).
4) Circulation for assisted wheelchair (negotiable width for corridors and doors).

The above can be interpreted as follows in terms of design:

1) Basically flat floor. No door sills, no step differences, unless vitally necessary.
2) Handrail installation at critical places, such as stairs, bathroom, toilet, and entrances.
3) Wider corridors and doors.
4) Gentler stairs.
5) Adoption of negotiable design features, such as door handles, water controls, electrical outlets, etc.
6) Preparedness for emergencies.

Some of the details have been modified since the author published a previous paper [9], but the basic ideas remain the same.

Issued Design Guidelines

The Design Guidelines were issued in June 1995 as two separate documents, one being issued by the Director-General of the Housing Bureau of the Ministry of Construction, the other by the Director of the Housing Construction and Improvement Division, the latter providing more detail (see Appendixes). The final Guidelines were based on the discussions of effectiveness, design and economic feasibility, climatic conditions, and cultural tradition. It has been the case in most countries to give due consideration to feasibility, climatic and cultural tradition when accessibility requirements are introduced, and Japan followed this course.

Implementation of Guidelines

Issuing guidelines does not ensure they will be put into practice. Japan has had a strong mechanism to force implementation, the Japan Housing Loan Corporation (HLC), a government organization for housing mortgages. HLC gives prospective clients lower interest rates for housing mortgages, and has been a driving force of Japan's economic growth. The Corporation took a decisive step in 1996 in making barrier-free or energy conscious designs eligible for the lowest interest rates. At the same time, the National Pension Housing Fund, a public organization affiliated with the Ministry of Health and Welfare, provided similar incentives for barrier-free designed homes. Along with the issuance of Guidelines, consumer education was provided through several approaches. With these steps taken, it was expected that their would be significant construction of barrier-free dwellings, and the majority of newer dwellings would be basically barrier-free in the long run (for more discussion from the viewpoint of housing policy, see [8]). For photos of a constructed house please refer to other papers [9][10].

There is clear evidence that these newer dwelling designs, in comparison of older designs, are well accepted by their residents [16] [18]. The introduction of the Guidelines was a significant success.

Now, about ten years later, what is the situation, and what needs to be done to further the movement toward promoting good design for older pepole?

Current Status

When the HLC introduced the new scheme of preferential interest rates in 1996, which required that either design for aging, energy conscious design or high durability design must be met, all the major housing providers adjusted their design standards to meet the new requirements (see Note). The actual perecentage of HLC housing mortgage usage related to design for older persons increased to more than 60 %, and Japanese residents accepted the concept of designing dwellings for ones' own future. This was followed by the introduction in 2000 of a housing performance indication system, based on the Housing Quality Assurance Law. Design for aging was included among the categories in the system [10] [11] [12].

A law on Securing Housing for Seniors was introduced in 2001. The primary goal was to invite the private rental sector into the housing market with economic incentives. The Design Guidelines of Dwellings for the Aged, revised version of the Design Guidelines of 1995, now became more formal than before.

Although the performance indication system is not mandatory, it is now gaining popularity because the trend is toward obtaining a long lasting dwelling rather than moving from one dwelling to another. People realize that keeping their property value in the long run is worthwhile, and that higher housing quality will appreciate more.

In 2004, around 3500 detached houses and 10,000 dwelling units within multi-family housing have a housing quality certificate. This means that the majority of newly built dwellings are without a certificate (roughly one million dwelling units are built in Japan every year), but there is a tendency toward applying for a certificate among multi-family housing units.

A certification system for existing dwellings was introduced in December 2002, but very few numbers of dwellings have applied thus far (127 detached houses and 89 multi-family dwellings as of March 2004). This is partly due to the cost/benefit ratio. It also relates to concern for the potential risk of exposing poorer quality and thus lowering the market value of the dwelling, particularly for multi-family units. Owners of other units do not want this to happen.

The introduction of a new law for securing housing for seniors was necessary because it is now impossible to accommodate all the seniors who wish to rent a public sector housing unit. The law introduced several economic benefits for private rental housing provision, from subsidies for construction, to assuring rents of seniors in cases of need. This is a change of emphasis from direct housing provision by the local governments, to encouraging, through incentives, private sector provision.

Whether this works effectively or not is yet to be seen because constructing new higher quality dwelling units targeted toward seniors could involve a large private sector investment. Existing dwelling units are generally of poor quality and normally it would be very expensive to modify them. For private banks that provide housing mortgages, higher quality dwellings are favored, which will help accelerate the trend toward design for ageing.

Regarding the official dwelling design guidelines for the aged, the content is quite similar to the previous design guidelines for the ageing society, which means that the contents of the guidelines are acceptable as the basis for all dwellings. The original 1995 Guidelines are included in the Appendicies.

Long-Term Care Insurance for the Aged

In April 2000, an insurance system that covers every senior citizen (in case of need) was introduced. It is managed by the Ministry of Health, Welfare and Labor, and was originally designed to assist seniors to age-in-place. Once an older person is certified to be in need of support due to frailty from aging, he/she is entitled to be supported in various ways, both physically and financially. However, the maximum amount one can receive to modify a dwelling is two hundred thousand yen, which is roughly two thousand US dollars. This amount is only enough for installation of handrails or something of the similar kind. Therefore, the system in reality denied effective home modifications to support seniors to continue to age-in-place.

The system instead allows quite a variety of assistive devices to be used (mostly rental), but is also generous for personal care assistance since the monthly cost to be covered for the above two kinds is in the same order of the maximum amount for home modification that is once-in-a-life-time. It seems that the Japanese Finance Ministry has a deep-rooted belief that housing provision should be done by the individuals. They feel that assisting elders with public money is social injustice. This is a rather different view from many other countries.

Assumed Residents in Dwellings

If aging-in-place is to be pursued, we must take it into consideration that the residents' capabilities can vary significantly. The official design guidelines of dwellings for the aged (and the HLC housing mortgage requirements) emphasized basically only the following three, i.e., floor without unnecessary level difference, support for handrail installation, and width of crucial space dimensions. These are not enough for more frail elders. However, in most cases additional arrangements can be provided if these three conditions are provided in advance [16]. Many of the difficulties encountered in the dwellings of the current frail seniors who wanted to be covered by the long-term care insurance system were related to the lack of the above three conditions, partly due to the old age of their dwellings [18]. Of course, if the residents have or develop severe disabilities, provisions to support their living in the dwellings (i.e., age-in-place) will have to be extensive and in some cases they need individualized solutions rather than generic, even if the dwellings are designed to match the aging of the residents. In many cases, however, the residents will be able to grow older without problems, as a resident survey demonstrated [18].

The baseline of Japanese design guidelines is far from desirable. What are needed for the future are: stricter requirements on stair dimensions, more dimension for circulation width, and solutions to level difference between outside and inside. The last issue is most difficult under climatic conditions of driving rain, and sophisticated methods in design and construction are necessary, particularly for detached houses.

In the global context, several facts are worth mentioning. In the UK (England and Wales), Approved Document Part M: Access and Facilities for Disabled People (1999 edition) requires that new residential construction must be accessible and usable on the ground floor (to include a bathroom on the ground floor). The visitability concept was originally introduced in the US (Atlanta, Georgia) in the late 1980s, and some local governments are trying to include the concept as requirements for new housing construction.

Conclusion

Existing dwellings are worse in terms of barrier-free design compared to newer ones. In addition, older persons who are more vulnerable and experiencing difficulties in their daily living tend to live in sub-standard dwellings with many barriers. To solve the problem, intervention at an earlier stage is desirable. Currently, there are few schemes that allow dwelling remodelling before residents develop difficulties or experience accidents during their daily activities. It is however necessary, from the viewpoint of ensuring QOL for older persons, to introduce a new scheme of financial assistance for remodelling. All we have now is a loan scheme from the Japan Housing Finance Agency. Unfortunately such loan schemes lack economic incentives for older residents even with some tax rebate. Japan must succeed in upgrading the quality of existing dwellings in a more effective way.

Acknowledgements

The author would like to express his sincere thanks to many colleagues in conducting experiments that provided the basis for the requirements of the design guidelines. The accomplishments were accepted because of such logical reasoning.

Notes

1. Although design for aging requirements did not lead to any serious problems, energy conscious design did. The simplest measure to meet energy saving requirement was to make the dwelling tight enough to prevent air from leaking, but it resulted in the so-called sick-house syndrome. To mitigate the problem, all dwellings are now legally required to have 24-hour ventilation system.

2. The Appendicies are the original Government Circular when the Design Guidelines were issued. There have been some minor changes after their issuance, yet the concept remained the same.

References

[1] Brink, S. (Ed) (1998). Housing Older People: An International Perspective. Transaction Publishers, New Brunswick, NJ.

[2] Department of the Environment, Transport and the Regions (1998). Approved document Part M: Access and Facilities for Disabled People; 1999 Edition (The Building Regulations). London, UK: The Stationery Office

[3] Kose, S. (1992). Capability of Daily Living of the Elderly and Their Accident Experiences: Implication to Design of Safer, Easier-to-Use Dwellings. In Equitable and Sustainable Habitats - Proceedings of EDRA23. EDRA, Oklahoma City, OK. 158-166.

[4] Kose, S. (1994). Housing for the Ageing Society: The Meaning of Barrier-free Design in Japan. MERA Journal. 2(1) 59-64. Kose, S. and Tanaka, Y. (2000). Dwelling Design for Seniors with Safety and Comfort in Mind. Tokyo: Ohm-sha. (in Japanese)

[5] Kose, S., Tanaka, Y., Suzuki, A. & Yamada, S. (1992c). Development of Technology for the Enhancement of Residential Environment in the Aging Society. In CIB92 Poster Book. Vol. 2, 424-425.

[6] National Research Institute for Population Problems (1986). 1986 Population Forecast.

[7] Salmen, J., Everyone's Welcome: The Americans with Disabilities Act and Museums. 1998, Washington, D.C.: American Association of Museums Bookstore.

[8] Kose, S. (1996). Possibilities for Change toward Universal Design: Japanese Housing Policy for Seniors at the Crossroads. Journal of Aging and Social Policy. 8(2&3) 161-176.

[9] Kose, S. (1997). Dwelling Design Guidelines for Accessibility in the Aging Society: A New Era in Japan? In Wapner S. et al, Eds., Handbook of Japan-US Environment Behavior Research: Toward a Transactional Approach, New York: Plenum. 25-42. Kose, S. (2001a). The Impact of Aging on Japanese Accessibility Standards. Preiser W. and Ostroff E. (Eds.), Universal Design Handbook. New York: McGraw-Hill. 17.1-17.12.

[10] Kose, S. (2001b). Design Guidelines of Dwellings for the Ageing Society: Japanese Approach Toward Universal Design. In CIB World Building Congress 2001 Proceedings, Wellington, NZ.

[11] Kose, S. (2003). The Japanese experience. Inclusive Design: Design for the whole population. London: Springer. 308-316.

[12] Kose, S. (2006) Universal Design of Dwellings: Who are the assumed residents? Gerontechnology, Vol. 5 No. 3, 170-173.

[13] Kose, S., Kumano, I., Ebara, K. & Kimura, D. (1992a). Physical Capabilities of Aged Persons Living as an Extended Family. In CIB92 Poster Book. Vol. 2. 422-423.

[14] Kose, S., Ohta, A., Tanaka, Y. & Watanabe, K. (1992b). Examination of Design Effectiveness of Special Housing for the Aged: Is Japanese "Silver-Housing" a Success? In Socio-Environmental Metamorphosis - Proceedings of IAPS12. Vol. 3. 161-166.

[15] Kose, S., Kumano, I. & Matsuzaki, A. (1999). How Far Has the Design of Dwellings Improved in These Ten Years?: Comparison of Two Groups of Houses from the Viewpoint of Design for the Ageing Society. In The Power of Imagination - Proceedings of EDRA30. EDRA, Edmond, OK. 127-132.

[16] Kose, S., Sugimoto, Y. & Goto, Y. (1991). Acceptable Handrail Position for Use by the Elderly. In Designing for Everyone - Proceedings of the Eleventh Congress of the International Ergonomics Association. 1116-1118.

Appendix 1. Design Guidelines for Dwellings in the Ageing Society (Government Circular by Director-General of Housing Bureau)
#67 HP/MOC 1995.06.23

To: Governors of Prefectures

From: Director-General, Housing Bureau, Ministry of Construction

RE: Design Guidelines for Dwellings in the Ageing Society

As we go into the 21st century, it is important to make it possible to continue to live safely in the community where the aged persons have lived so far. To accomplish the goal, new housing construction shall be designed and made from the beginning to allow for the residents to continue to live their daily life, should they develop physical and functional deterioration or disabilities due to ageing, etc.

From the social welfare policy viewpoint, more extensive care-giving at home is the critical issues and it is most important for dwelling design to give due consideration for their fulfilment.

To attain the goal, and to promote public education based on the concept of the Law on Building Accessible and Usable Buildings by Aged and Disabled Persons (No. 44/1994), the following design guidelines of dwellings for the ageing society (DG) have been finally established. I hereby send the DG as my duty.

I strongly suggest that you will understand the purpose and ideas of DG. I also ask you to try to do within your capacity to enforce the DG in the dwelling design for PORH, RH/PH by your Local Housing Associations, etc. I also urge you to send the DG to transmit to Local Governments, Housing Associations, Association of Regional Architects, etc.

1. General:

1-1 Purpose

The Guidelines intend to give guidance on how to design dwellings that will allow residents to continue to live in the same dwelling even if they develop problems of functional capability deterioration or disability, thereby promoting constructing dwellings suited to the aged society.

1-2 Scope (Coverage)

(1) The guidelines mainly apply to new construction, including

replacement of old dwellings.
(2) The guidelines refer to general ideas of dwelling design only. If one intends to give individual considerations to residents who already developed physical and functional deterioration or disabilities, it will be necessary, in some cases, to take into account of other ideas in addition to those described here.
(3) The guidelines will be revised as social context changes and technical developments come up.

2. Design Guidelines of Respective Dwellings (or dwelling units for multifamily dwellings)
2-1 General (Common) Requirements
(1) Layout of spaces
(a) The following rooms/spaces are to be on the same floor level if possible: Entrance, toilet, washroom, bathroom, dressing room, living room, dining room, and aged person's (AP) bedroom.
(b) Toilet, washroom, living room and dining room shall be closely located with AP bedroom, if possible.
(c) In the DG, the AP bedroom means a room that is normally expected to be used as such in the future.
(d) If there will be multiple rooms/spaces in a dwelling, at least one of each shall follow the DG.

2-1-2 Level differences
Internal floors shall be level, without step differences, door sills, etc. However, main entrance, and level differences for taking off shoes area, entrance to bathroom area, and entrance to outside balconies can have thresholds.

2-1-3 Handrails
(a) Stairs and bathroom shall have handrails.
(b) Entrance, toilet, washroom, dressing room, living room and dining room, aged person's bedroom, and corridor, etc., shall have handrails, either from the beginning or with later installation.
(c) Handrails shall be of usable shape and materials, and shall be installed at appropriate locations and height.

2-1-4 Width of corridor and doors
Width of corridors and doors shall be made to allow for smooth passage of walking-aids and assisted wheelchairs.

2-1-5 Floor/wall finishes
Finishes of internal floors and walls shall be safe against

slipping, collision, and falls.

2-1-6 Doors/sliding partitions, etc. (openings)
Openings shall be safe and easily usable. The operating devices (grips, handles, locking devices) shall be usable and be properly located.

2-1-7 Building appliances
(a) Water and hot water supply, electrical appliances, and gas appliances shall be safe and easily operable.
(b) Lighting appliances be properly located for safety, and sufficient lighting shall be provided.
(c) Fire alarms and emergency reporting systems shall be provided, or shall be prepared for later installation.

2-1-8 Thermal environment
Environmental design (insulation and ventilation) shall be such that temperature difference between rooms/spaces be minimized. It is expected that heating/cooling equipment be installable, to maintain proper temperature all year round.

2-1-9 Storage
Storage space for daily use shall be properly provided. It shall be easily usable without requiring difficult posture.

2-2 Internal spaces
2-2-1 Main entrance
(a) Level difference at the main entrance shall be safe.
(b) Space for entrance shall be wide enough to have a seat available.
(c) Level difference between shod and unshod areas shall be easily manageable height, with intermediate steps where needed.

2-2-2 Stairs
Stair pitch and shape shall be safe for ascent and descent.

2-2-3 Toilet
(a) Toilet shall be provided with enough floor area for care-giving, if possible.
(b) Entrance to toilet shall be made not to hinder emergency assistance (including unlocking).
(c) Toilet shall be of sitting type (not be of squatting type).

2-2-4 Washroom/Dressing room
(a) Washroom shall be designed for the ease of hand washing,

etc.
(b) Dressing room shall be designed for the safety of clothing/unclothing.

2-2-5 Bathroom
(a) Bathroom shall have enough space for care-giving, if possible.
(b) Should there be level differences between bathroom and dressing room, it shall be safely designed, and handrails shall be provided.
(c) Doors of the bathroom entrance shall be safely designed, as well as designed for emergency assistance (including helping someone out).
(d) Bathtub shall be of such shape and dimension designed for safety.

2-2-6 Aged person's bedroom
Aged person's bedroom shall be wide enough to allow for potential care-giving. It shall be designed with sound insulation and emergency evacuation in mind.

2-2-7 Balconies, etc.
Level differences at the balconies shall be designed to give due consideration to safety.

3. Design guide for external space for multi-family dwellings
3-1 Approaches, etc.
(a) Main circulation within the housing blocks and main entrance to a building block shall be designed with safety and usability of walking-aids and wheelchairs.
(b) Entrance of the block shall be accessible by cars, and parking space shall be provided if possible.

3-2 Public stairs
Public stairs shall be designed with safety in mind, in particular for pitch and shape.

3-3 Public corridor/circulation
Public corridor shall be provided with enough width for wheelchair maneuvering, where possible, and no level differences shall be allowed.

3-4 Floor finishes and handrail provisions
(a) Floor finishes of approaches, entrance to the building block,

stairs, ramps and corridors shall be designed with safety against slipping and tripping in mind.
(b) Stairs, ramps, and corridors shall be provided with handrails.
(c) Handrails shall be of usable shape and materials, and shall be installed at appropriate locations.

3-5 Elevators
(a) Block of dwelling units with six stories and higher shall have elevators. Blocks with three to five stories shall have elevators if possible.
(b) Circulation and the block entrance to elevator hall, and elevator hall, and elevator cage shall be designed to allow for wheelchair accessibility (shape, and dimension).

3-6 Lighting appliances
Lighting for external approaches and common spaces shall be properly done with safety in mind.

4 Design guide for external space of detached houses
4-1 Approaches, etc.
(a) Approach circulation shall be designed to accommodate for walking-aids and wheelchair use (shape and dimension).
(b) External stairs shall be designed with safety in mind, in particular for pitch and shape.
(c) Enough external lighting level shall be provided with safety in mind.

Appendix 2. Design Guidelines for Dwellings in the Ageing Society (Government Circular by Director of Housing Construction and Improvement Division) #68 HP/MOC 1995.06.23

To: Directors of Housing Department

From: Director of Housing Construction and Improvement, Housing Bureau, MOC

Re: Supplementary guidelines to DG

While DG have been sent as #63, this document is intended to supplement DG for more productive utilization as regards to dimensions, specifications, etc.

DG and the current Supplementary DG aim at providing

ageing in place with reasonable provisions for supporting physical deterioration expected to come with ageing (i.e., use of sticks, walking aids etc., for independent living), and support for assisted wheelchair living.

Some of the requirements include additional features to increase safety and comfort or to have more usable design with wheelchairs, which are optional with economic or space conditions.

The DG supplement is expected to be revised as social context changes and technological developments come up.

I. Inside of dwelling units

1. General

(1) Room/space layout

- As regards the requirement having rooms/spaces on the same floor level, it is acceptable to have a room/space (on the same floor level) that can be convertible (with minor adaptations, for example partitioning) to suite for the purpose if need arises.
- AP bedroom and toilet shall be on the same floor level, but other room/space does not have to be, provided that the space/room be reachable with installation of a home elevator or a stair lift (installation afterward is acceptable).

(2) Level differences

Raised or lowered room/space such as an extra room, tatami corner in the main living room, which are away from main circulation of AP daily activities, and no use by AP is expected, can have level differences.

(3) Handrails

Stairs shall have handrails at least on one side, and there shall be provisions for future installation on the other side. (i.e., strong enough to support).

- End of stair handrails shall be extended horizontally 20 cm or longer as much as possible, unless they are continuously installed with the rails of the corridor, etc.
- Handrails for going in/out of a bathtub shall be installed. There shall also be a handrail at the entrance to bathroom as much as possible.
- There shall be a handrail, or provisions for later installation, at the level difference of the entrance hall in order to assist putting on/off shoes.
- Handrails shall be provided or prepared for later installation of toilet in order to assist sitting down/standing up and securing posture.
- Dressing room shall have handrails or prepare for later

installation to assist changing clothes.

- Standard height of handrails to be installed for movement at corridor, stairs, washroom, living/dining room, AP room shall be 75 cm from the floor (as with stairs, the height be measure at the nosing).
- End of horizontal handrails be turned to the wall or down side.
- Recommended:
- Handrails better be provided on both sides of stairs.
- Bathroom shall have handrails that assist sitting down/ standing up in the bathtub, in the washing area, and to secure posture.

(4) Width of corridor and doors

- Effective width of corridors shall be 78 cm or wider (if there exist columns etc., 75 cm width is acceptable for such part).
- Door effective width (to be measure excluding door thickness for swing doors, excluding projecting part for sliding doors) shall be 75 cm or wider. For bathroom doors, 65 cm (or 60 cm if it is definitely unavoidable) is acceptable. Doors other than the ones for main entrance and bathrooms can be less than the required width, if it is unavoidable but reasonable provision is done for remodeling afterwards.
- For the corner of corridor, or corridor that is next to an entrance needing turning approach, there shall be a space that allows turning of assisted wheelchair. The space could be remodeled afterwards.
- Recommended:
- Effective width of corridors shall be 85 cm or wider (if there exist columns etc., 80 cm width is acceptable for such part).
- Effective door width shall be 80 cm or wider.

(5) Floor/wall finish

- Floor shall be finished to be non-slippery. Reasonable measures shall be provided to reduce impact when there is a fall. Bathroom floor is most slippery that special care shall be made.
- Stair tread shall be non-skid finish or provided with non-slip.
- Corner of corridors shall be given due consideration for shape and finish, such as rounding, against collision.

(6) Doors/sliding partition, etc. (openings)

- If the entrance is a swing door, devices such as door closers shall be installed to prevent abrupt opening/closing.

- Locks of bathroom and toilet doors shall be unlockable from the outside in case of emergency.
- If doors are glazed, safety glasses shall be used, or the dimension of glazing shall be limited.
- Recommended
- Side wall of 30cm or wider shall be provided on the swing/ opening side of doors.
- Entrance door shall be double leaf (effective width of main leaf shall be 80cm minimum).
- Glasses of doors, windows and fixed furniture shall be safety glazing if they have potential of contact with humans.

(7) Appliances

- Faucets shall be easily operable (such as lever type), as well as temperature controlled for safety against scalds.
- Switches and electric outlets shall be placed at easily operable height. They shall be large and easily noticeable with indicators as much as possible.
- Lighting for stairs shall be installed to prevent dark spots occurring during use. The switches shall be operable from both ends of stairs.
- Gas appliances shall be safe against leakage of unburned gas due to accidental fire blow out, etc.
- Gas leak detector and fire alarm shall be installed in the kitchen. Emergency alarm system shall be installed at the toilet and bathroom as much as possible.
- Recommended
- Footlights shall be installed for stairs.
- Footlights shall be installed at the level difference of the entrance.
- Automatic fire extinguishers or sprinklers shall be installed at the kitchen.
- Emergency alarm systems shall be installed for the aged persons' room.

(8) Thermal environment

- Heating appliances shall be installed or prepared for installation at the toilet, washroom, dressing room, living/ dining room and aged persons' room. Cooling appliances shall be prepared for installation at living/dining room and aged persons' room according to the climatic conditions.
- Heating appliances shall be installed at bathroom according to climatic conditions.

2. Inside dwelling units

(1) Entrance

- Level difference between door sills and outside shall be 2cm maximum. Level difference between door sill and inside shall be 5mm maximum.
- Level difference between shod area and unshod area at the entrance shall be 11cm maximum for dwelling units of multi-family housing, and 18cm maximum for detached houses. If it is not possible to comply, intermediate steps shall be installed or prepared for installation to make height difference between steps shall be 18cm or less.
- The level difference at the entrance shall be clearly visible, with change in materials texture, colour, etc.
- Recommended
- Level difference at the entrance shall be eliminated.

(2) Stairs

- Stair pitch shall be 6/7 maximum, and relationship between tread and rise shall comply with the equation of $55<2R+T<65$ (cm). If the above is not possible, pitch shall be 22/21 maximum, $T>19.5$cm, and $55<2R+T<65$. Handrail shall be installed on both sides if the pitch exceeds 45 degrees.
- Intrusion of first/last steps to circulation spaces shall be avoided. Winding stairs shall be avoided as much as possible.
- If non-skid nosing is used, it shall be made flat with the rest of tread surface as much as possible. Stair risers shall be installed, and nosing overhang shall be avoided as much as possible. Maximum overhang of tread shall be 2cm (3cm if it is unavoidable).
- Recommended
- Stair pitch shall be 7/11 maximum, with $55<2R+T<65$.

(3) Toilet

- Space for assisting toilet activities shall be provided or prepared for provision, as much as possible.
- Recommended
- Dimension of toilet shall be 1.35m wide and 1.35m depth.

(4) Washroom/dressing room

- Recommended
- Wash basin that allows usage with chair shall be installed.
- Pre-washing sink shall be installed at the dressing room (or near washing machine).

(5) Bathroom

Bathroom shall be wide enough to allow usage of bathing chair. It shall be 2.5 sqm minimum with narrower dimension being 1.4m minimum. If this is not possible, 1.8 sqm with narrower dimension 1.2m for multi-family dwelling unit, or 2.0 sqm with narrower dimension 1.3m is permitted.

- Level difference at the entrance to bathroom shall be 2cm maximum. If it is not possible, maximum height difference between lower side and door sill shall be 18cm, height difference between inside and outside shall be 12cm. In this case, handrail shall be installed.
- Entrance door shall be a sliding or folding door. If a door which swings inside is used, it shall be designed to be detachable from the outside in case of emergency.
- Height of bathtub from the washing area shall be between 30cm and 50cm.
- Recommended
- Level difference at the entrance shall be eliminated.
- Edge of bathtub shall be designed to allow for sitting on it.
- Height of bathtub from the washing area shall be between 35cm and 45cm.

(6) Aged persons' room

- Aged persons' room shall be 12 sqm or larger. If this is not possible, it shall be 10 sqm.

(7) Balcony, etc.

- Level difference at the entrance to outside balcony/terrace shall be 18cm without upstand. If this is not possible, 25cm height difference without upstand or maximum 18cm upstand on both sides. For these cases, handrail shall be installable.
- Height of clothes hanger shall be designed for use by the aged persons as much as possible.
- Recommended
- For multi-family housing, emergency evacuation route to the next dwelling unit shall be designed to be easily operable.

II. Common space for multi-family housing

1. Approach, etc.

- External pedestrian circulation shall be minimum 90 cm wide, with intermittent wider spaces. Ramps shall be introduced as much as possible if there is difference in level.
- External stairs shall be designed as R<16 cm and T>30 cm. If it is unavoidable, T>24 cm with 55<T+2R<65 is permitted.
- Pitch of ramps shall be maximum 1/12 as much as possible, and ramps shall have horizontal landings of 1.5 m going at every 75 cm height difference.
- Recommended
- Eternal pedestrian circulation shall have 120 cm minimum

width.

2. Public stairs

- Public stairs shall have 120 cm effective width as much as possible, maximum pitch 7/11, $55<T+2R<65$. If it is unavoidable, $T>24$ cm with $55<T+2R<65$ is permitted. In the case where usual vertical circulation is covered by elevators and the public stairs are only used for emergencies, the above requirement does not apply.
- Public stairs shall be designed so that intrusion of first/last steps to circulation spaces will be avoided. The stair shape shall be straight or dogleg with landings, as much as possible.
- If non-skid nosing is used, it shall be made flat with the rest of tread surface as much as possible. Stair risers shall be installed, and nosing overhang shall be avoided as much as possible. Maximum overhang of tread shall be 2cm (3cm if it is unavoidable).
- Recommended
- Public stairs shall be designed as $R<16$ cm, $T>30$ cm.

3. Public corridor

Effective width of public corridor shall be minimum 140 cm as much as possible, and spaces for pass-by of wheelchairs shall be introduced at places.

- Public corridor side of main entrance door of dwelling units shall have alcove as much as possible.

4. Surface finish and handrails

- Stairs and ramps shall have handrails at least on one side. The end shall be extended horizontally minimum 20 cm as much as possible.
- Public corridor shall have handrails at least on one side.
- The height of handrails shall be 75 cm standard, and the end shall be turned to wall or down side as much as possible.
- Recommended
- Stairs and ramps shall have handrails on both sides.

5. Elevator

- If there exists level difference between entrance to the building block and elevator lobby, both stairs and ramps shall be provided as much as possible. Their effective width shall be 120 cm minimum.
- Elevator lobby shall have enough space for wheelchair

turning (150 cm square), and the entrance door of the elevator shall be 80 cm minimum.

- Elevator call button and operating switches shall be designed for use by people with wheelchairs.
- Recommended
- Elevators shall be installed for two storied building block.
- Elevator cage shall be 135 cm deep minimum, 2 sqm minimum, and shall have extended storage apace.

6. Lighting appliances

- Lighting of public stairs shall be designed to avoid shadow formation during use (for example multiple lamps).
- Recommended
- Public stairs shall have foot lights.

III. Design of external space for detached houses

1. Approach, etc.

- If there is a level difference in the land lot, shallow stairs or ramps shall be provided, with handrails at least on one side.
- If stairs are to be provided, stairs of a few steps from the public road into the land lot shall be $R<16$ cm, $T>30$ cm. Other stairs shall be $T<24$ cm, $55<T+2R<65$.
- Lighting for external stairs shall be designed to avoid shadow formation during use.
- Recommended
- Level difference at approach shall have foot lights.

Aging, Disability and Independence
W.C. Mann (Ed.)
IOS Press, 2008

doi:10.3233/978-1-58603-902-8-41

Accessible Design Practices and Informal Learning Environments

Carrie Bruce[1] and Elizabeth Bryant[1]
[1]Center for Assistive Technology and Environmental Access (CATEA) at Georgia Institute of Technology

Abstract: Informal learning environments, such as aquaria, are attracting an increasingly diverse visitor population as the number of people with disabilities living in the community has grown. Although general guidelines exist to assist informal learning environments in designing accessible spaces, the guidelines are not specific enough nor do they guarantee that the spaces will be usable by all visitors. This paper reports on the findings from a post-occupancy evaluation that was conducted at the Georgia Aquarium that: 1) documented the current exhibit display and interpretation design practices; 2) provided visitor feedback on the usability of exhibit displays and interpretation; and 3) discussed the needs of visitors with disabilities.

Keywords: informal learning environments, ILEs, aquaria, exhibit design, interpretation, accessibility, accessible design, museums, zoos

Introduction

Among the common goals of informal learning environments (ILEs), including aquaria, are the education and entertainment of the visiting public. However, as the number of people with disabilities living in the community has grown, and as public environments have become more accessible to them, ILEs are faced with educating an increasingly diverse visitor population with varying physical and sensory needs. Although ADA Accessibility Guidelines (ADAAG) [1] have improved facility access, these requirements are primarily intended to facilitate physical access for people who use wheelchairs [2] [3] and even then, are too general to apply directly to exhibit design [4]. Other field publications [5] [6] [7]have been produced to respond to the lack of guidance that would enable ILEs to provide more accessible exhibit displays and interpretation. However, these guidelines lack specific direction on how to determine which design characteristics will work best for a particular setting or specific types of exhibits within an ILE.

The first step toward identifying effective design practices for aquarium exhibit displays and interpretation that meets the needs of visitors with disabilities is to better understand the barriers and facilitators that are experienced. As the majority of the information on effectiveness of design practices in ILEs related to individuals with disabilities is anecdotal and provides minimal contribution for supporting existing practices or aiding in improved design criteria of exhibits, this study sought to evaluate exhibit features and characteristics that were either barriers or facilitators for visitors with disabilities.

This paper reports on the findings from a post-occupancy evaluation that was conducted at the Georgia Aquarium to inform on effectiveness of current exhibit design by: 1) documenting the current exhibit display and interpretation design practices used at the Georgia Aquarium; 2) providing visitor feedback on the usability of exhibit displays and interpretation; and 3) discussing the needs of visitors with disabilities. The resulting practice assessment data will be used to guide future research, and eventually, development of improved design of exhibits that incorporates the needs of visitors with disabilities.

Methods

Post-occupancy evaluation involves systematic evaluation of how a building meets the needs of the users. This type of evaluation is an effective process for generating information that provides experiential feedback that is useful in development of future research and design. This evaluation was conducted through touring interviews and focus groups with individuals with various disabilities.

Participants

Twenty-nine adults (15 males and 14 females) were recruited through local organizations involved in disability service provision. The participants each had at least one functional limitation, including impairments in vision, motor, hearing, speech, and cognition. Participants ranged in age from 24 to 80 years old, with a mean age of 48 years. Subjects were divided into 10 groups, with eight groups arranged homogeneously according to primary functional limitation: blindness, low vision, hard of hearing, deafness, motor impairment, cognitive impairment, and speech impairment. Two additional heterogeneous groups were comprised of individuals having vision, motor, speech, and/or hearing impairments. Each group visited two pre-identified galleries for the touring interviews and then participated in a

Table 1. Features and Characteristics of Exhibits

Features	Characteristics

Display
The animal(s), and the habitat or immediate environment of the animal.
	• **Position**
	  ○ Viewing height: the height at which the animal can be viewed.
	  ○ Interaction height: the height at which the animal can be touched.
	  ○ Distance: the how far away the display and its contents are, given that the visitor is as close as possible.
	• **Lighting:** the natural or artificial lighting inside the display.
	• **Visibility:** whether the display is visibly apparent and whether its contents can be seen, given the opacity/transparency of the display materials and the density of display contents.

Interpretation
The descriptive or informational detail typically presented in *static* (delivery of "canned" facts) or *dynamic* (interactive and flexible content and style of delivery) formats through techniques such as signage, kiosks, recorded video, docents, and/or recorded audio.
	• **Position**
	  ○ Viewing height: the height at which the interpretation can be viewed.
	  ○ Interaction height: the height at which the interpretation can be touched, activated, or controlled.
	  ○ Distance: the how far away the interpretation is, given that the visitor is as close as possible.
	  ○ Proximity: the distance the interpretation is from the display.
	  ○ Angle: the slant of the interpretation from the horizontal or vertical plane.
	• **Lighting:** the natural or artificial lighting behind, in front of, or to the side that is meant to illuminate the interpretation.
	• **Visibility:** whether the interpretation is visibly apparent and whether its information can be seen, given the opacity/transparency of the interpretation materials.
	• **Readability**
	  ○ Speed: the timing of interpretation or the amount of time before the interpretation changes.
	  ○ Font size/type: letters/characters height, width, and style.
	  ○ Color/contrast: the color or tone combination that makes the text distinguishable from the background.
	  ○ Finish: surface texture or appearance.
	• **Graphics:** drawings, pictures, and other non-textual content.
	• **Information sufficiency:** the quantity, depth, and relevancy of information presented.
	• **Sound**
	  ○ Speed: rate at which tones or speech is presented.
	  ○ Gender: the male of female quality of the speech.
	  ○ Loudness: the intensity of the sound.

Surrounding Environment
The features and characteristics in the space around exhibits
	• **Lighting:** the natural or artificial lighting that is in the surrounding area of the exhibit.
	• **Path**
	  ○ Flooring: type, texture, and reflectivity of the surface.
	  ○ Elevation changes: steps in or slope of the surface.
	  ○ Width: the side-to-side passage distance in front of or around exhibit.
	  ○ Color/contrast: the color or tone combination of the surface.
	• **Ambient sound:** the type and loudness of sounds (non-crowd) in the surrounding area.
	• **Fixtures and furnishings**
	  ○ Physical dimensions: the height, length, width, etc. that affects how a visitor is able to interact with or use the fixture/furnishing.
	  ○ Obstructions: physical barriers preventing view, interaction, or use.
	• **Crowd**
	  ○ Sound: the noise produced by the crowd.
	  ○ Navigation: the density and flow of the crowd in front of or around the exhibit that impacts traveling.
	  ○ Viewing: the density or height of the crowd in front of or around the exhibit that impacts viewing.

focus group. Twenty subjects' comments were recorded during the touring interview to collect more detailed information. All 29 subjects participated in the focus groups after visiting the galleries.

Independent Variables

Description of displays, interpretation, and the surrounding environment involved systematically documenting each exhibit in the five galleries of the Georgia Aquarium. The process of categorizing exhibit features and characteristics is based on an analysis of a broad range of exhibit displays and interpretation from over 30 aquaria, zoos, art and cultural museums, and science centers around the United States and Canada. (See Table 1)

Procedure

To evaluate the unique barriers and needs that visitors with disabilities experienced with exhibit displays at the Georgia Aquarium, this project included two phases: 1) site documentation: the description of exhibit displays and interpretation; and 2) visitor evaluation: evaluation of exhibit display and interpretation through touring interviews and focus groups.

Site Documentation. The investigators visited the aquarium several times at the start of the study to review all exhibits according to the independent variables mentioned previously. Photographs were taken and observation of general visitors was performed to enable the investigators to become familiar with exhibit features and characteristics.

Visitor Evaluation. Exhibit features and characteristics were evaluated through two methods that gathered input from individuals with disabilities: 1) touring interviews and 2) focus groups. The touring interviews involved groups of two to four people and were completed with only 20 of the subjects. Each study group visited two of the five galleries, with each gallery being visited by two different study groups. All data was classified according to the previously mentioned taxonomy.

Results

Barriers. Touring Interview Within Exhibit Analysis. The data revealed that three exhibits (out of 38), Cold Water Quest touch tank, River Scout Electric Fish, and Tropical Diver Coral Reef, had the highest number of reported barriers, accounting for 30%

(n=43) of the total number of comments (n=147) about problems with exhibit access.

The Cold Water Quest touch tank exhibit had 21 comments related to barriers. Almost half of the comments (n=10) were related to the interaction and viewing height of the display. Position and readability of printed signs, sound of the crowd, and ambient sounds were mentioned as barriers four times. Physical access to fixtures and furnishings were stated as barriers in three instances. Individuals with motor impairments had problems with display viewing height (n=5), display interaction height (n=5), and fixtures and furnishings (n=3). Individuals with hearing impairments had problems with ambient sound and sound of the crowd (n=2), and the position of the printed sign (n=2). Individuals with vision impairments had difficulty with the position and readability of printed signs (n=2). Individuals with speech impairments mentioned ambient sound and sound of the crowd (n=2) as barriers.

The River Scout Electric Fish exhibit had 11 comments associated with it. Position of the printed signs and video caption were the most frequently cited barriers, being referred to in over half of the cases (n=7). In addition, problems with the viewing height of the display, readability of the printed sign, fixtures and furnishings, and sound of video (loudness) were each reported once. Individuals with motor impairments reported over 73% of the barriers (n=8) for this exhibit, indicating problems with position of printed signs and video (n=5), viewing height of the display (n=1), sound of video (loudness) (n=1), and fixtures and furnishings (obstruction) (n=1). Individuals with hearing impairments mentioned position of video (n=2) and readability of printed sign (n=1).

Tropical Diver's Coral Reef exhibit was commented on 11 times. The readability of the kiosks and the video monitor signs were mentioned on five occasions. There were four other comments related to kiosks, including two concerning position and information sufficiency, one that was categorized as interactivity of kiosk (i.e., not having the strength to activate the kiosk), and one categorized as visibility of interpretation (i.e., not knowing the kiosk was there or what it did). Two comments related to visibility of display contents were also noted. Individuals with vision impairments cited issues with readability of printed signs, kiosks, and video monitor signs

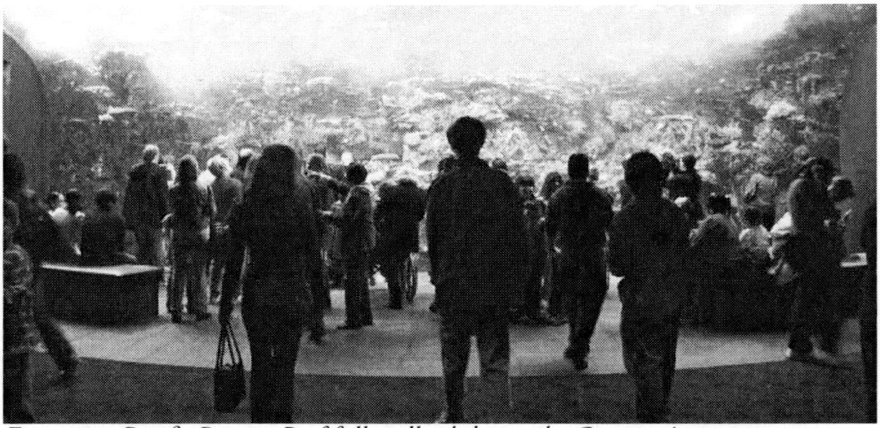

Figure 1 – Pacific Barrier Reef full wall exhibit at the Georgia Aquarium.

(n=5) and position of kiosk (n=1). Participants in this group also provided comments related to visibility of display and kiosk (n=2) and interaction height of interpretation (n=1). Information sufficiency of kiosk (hearing impairment; n=1) and position of kiosk (motor impairment; n=1) also presented barriers.

Touring Interview Across Exhibits Analysis. The features and characteristics that individuals commented on the most were position of the printed signs (n=26), viewing height of the display (n=20), visibility of display contents (n=11), lighting for printed signs (n=11), visibility of display contents (n=11), and readability of printed signs (n=10). Position of printed signs included viewing height (n=17), proximity (n=7), distance (n=1), and angle (n=1). Comments for lighting of printed signs referred to brightness (n=9) and glare (n=2). Readability of printed signs included comments on font size and style (n=4), "other" (overall readability) (n=3), and contrast (n=3).

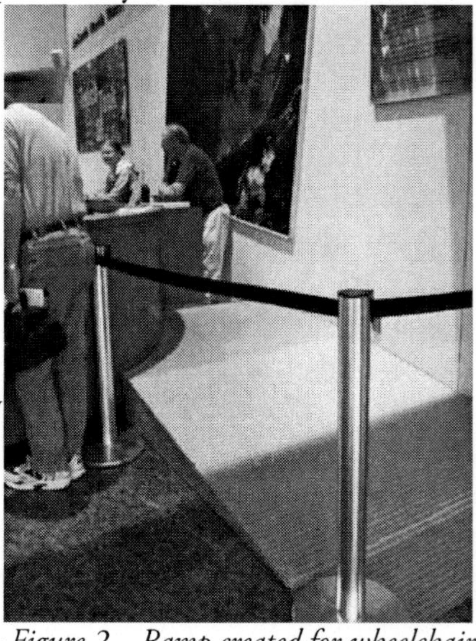

Figure 2 – Ramp created for wheelchair access to touch tank at the Florida Aquarium

Individuals with motor impairments represented the only group to experience barriers with viewing height of display (n=20) and offered the greatest number of comments about the viewing height of printed signs (n=15). These individuals also experienced barriers with lighting of printed

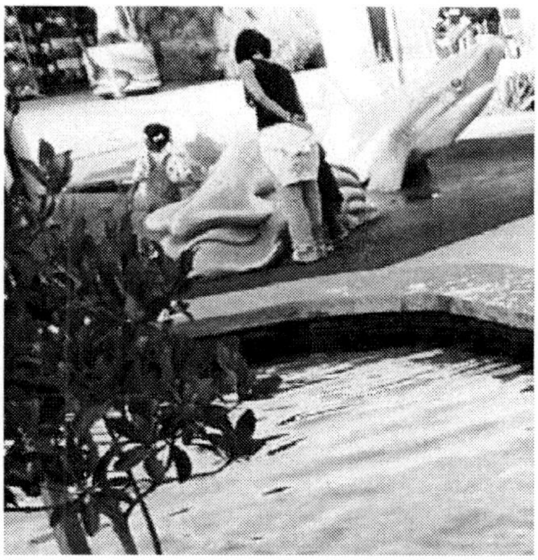

Figure 3 – Touch tank with wall at lower height at the Aquarium of the Pacific.

signs (n=4) and readability of printed signs (n=2). Individuals with vision impairments provided the only comments related to visibility of display contents (n=11) and the greatest number for lighting of printed signs (n=5) and readability of printed signs (n=6). This group also stated problems with position of printed signs (n=5). Individuals with hearing impairments experienced issues with position (n=2), lighting (n=2), and readability (n=2) of printed signs.

Focus Group Results. The four features and characteristics that represented the greatest number of comments about barriers during the focus groups were crowd issues (n=11), general information sufficiency (n=8), position of video (n=7), and fixtures and furnishings (n=7). Crowd issues were related to sound (n=4), navigation (n=4), and viewing (n=3) problems. Position of video comments were associated with viewing height (n=5) and interaction height (n=2). Barriers with fixtures and furnishings were noted according to physical access (to hand washing) (n=3), obstructions, (n=2), and seating (n=2).

Although greater than half (n=42) of the total number of comments (n=83) were mentioned by individuals with motor impairments, individuals with vision impairments averaged five comments per participant (compared to 3.8 for motor, 1.7 for cognitive, 1.5 for hearing, and .5 for speech). Individuals with

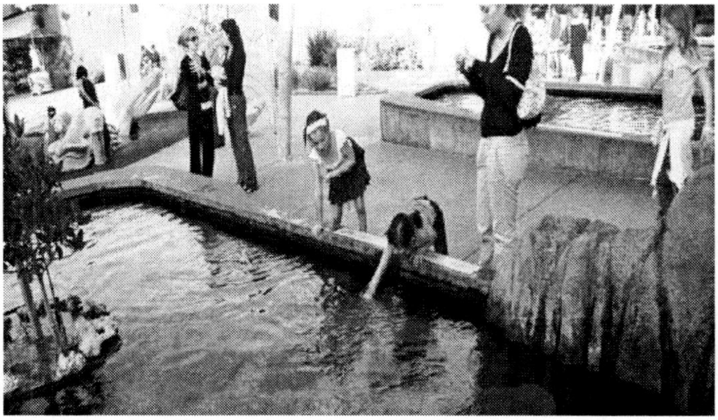

Figure 4 – Touch tank that is narrow and shallow at the Aquarium of the Pacific

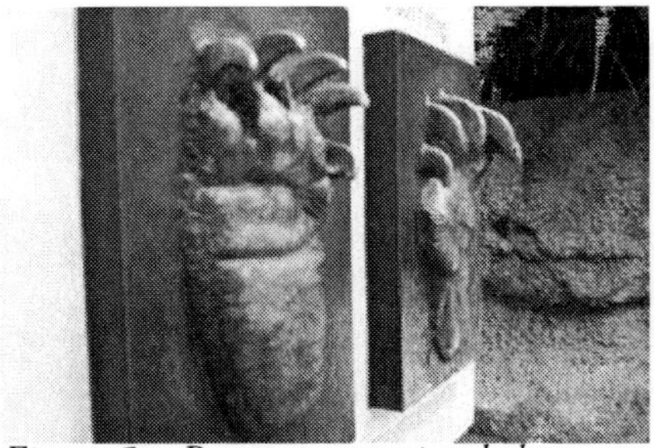

Figure 5 – Bronze cast animal claws at the San Diego Zoo.

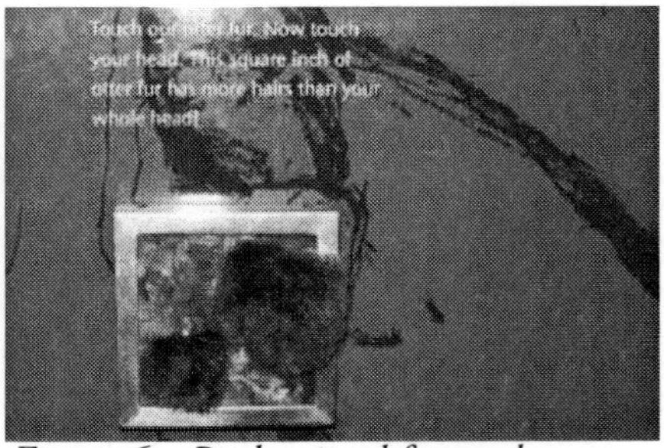

Figure 6 – Real animal fur at the Aquarium of the Pacific.

motor impairments made comments in 76% (n=16) of the exhibit features and characteristics that were discussed in the focus groups, with the greatest issues in viewing height of display (n=4), interaction height of display (n=4), and general information sufficiency (n=4). Individuals with vision impairments experienced problems with 72% (n=15) of the exhibit features and characteristics, noting the majority of barriers in general information sufficiency (n=3), lighting (n=3), and floor plan/map (n=3). Individuals in the hearing, cognitive, and speech groups mentioned fewer barriers. The hearing group provided comments related to 28% (n=6) of the features and characteristics and stated the greatest number of barriers in graphics on printed signs (n=3), the cognitive group stated problems with 24% (n=5), and the speech group mentioned issues with 10% (n=1).

Facilitators. Touring Interview Within Exhibit Analysis. During the touring interviews, participants also provided positive feedback about the usability of design features and characteristics of exhibits. The data suggested that participants had the greatest number of positive comments (n=9) related to the Arawana and

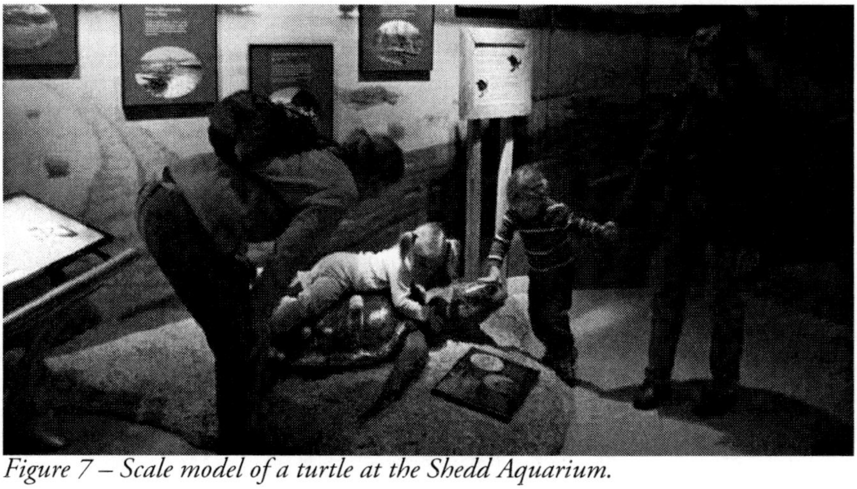

Figure 7 – Scale model of a turtle at the Shedd Aquarium.

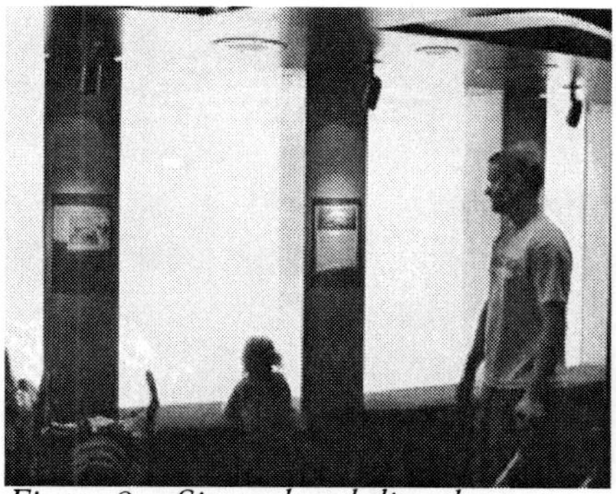

Figure 8 – Signs placed directly next to viewing windows at Vancouver Aquarium

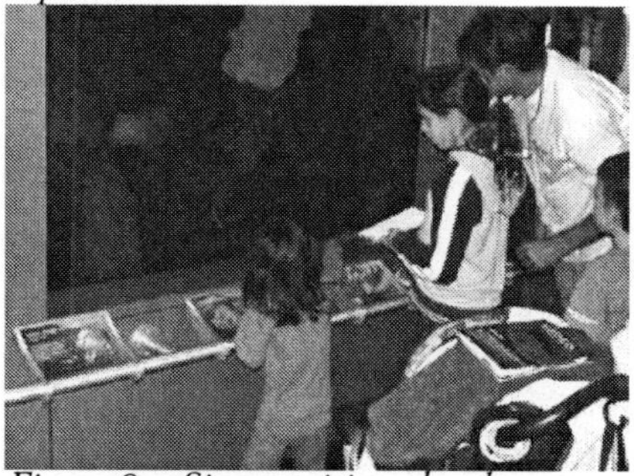

Figure 9 – Signs positioned at lower height at the Aquarium of the Pacific.

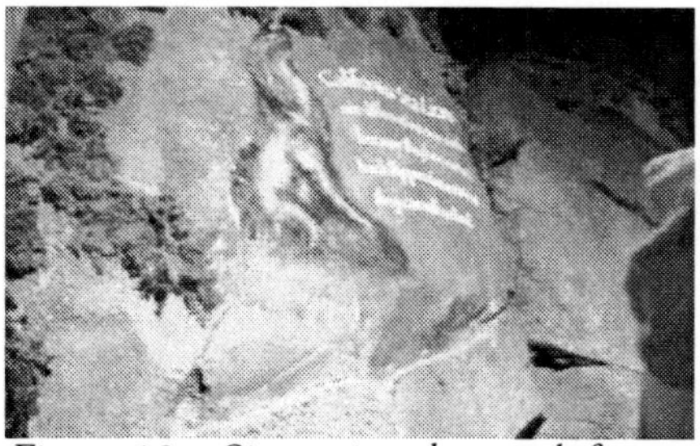

Figure 10 – Sign painted on rock face at the Sea Lions exhibit at the Georgia Aquarium.

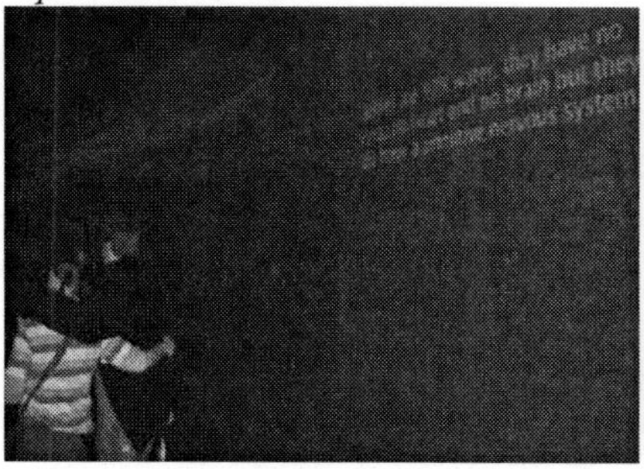

Figure 11 – Projected sign on wall at Jellies exhibit at the Georgia Aquarium.

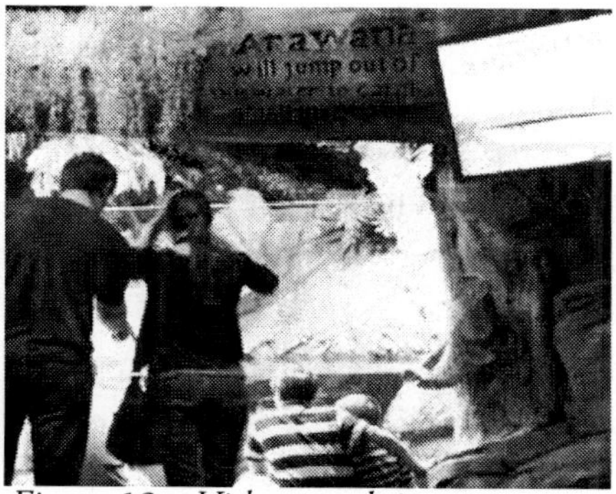

Figure 12 – Video panel signs at Arawana/Arapaima at the Georgia Aquarium.

Arapaima exhibit in River Scout. This exhibit had three comments related to the readability of the video sign, three related to information sufficiency of the video sign, and three comments that were categorized as “other” referring to liking the video signs. Individuals with motor impairments provided the most positive comments (n=8) about this exhibit’s features and characteristics, experiencing facilitators in all of the categories for video signs as previously mentioned.

Touring Interview Across Exhibits Analysis. The features and characteristics that produced

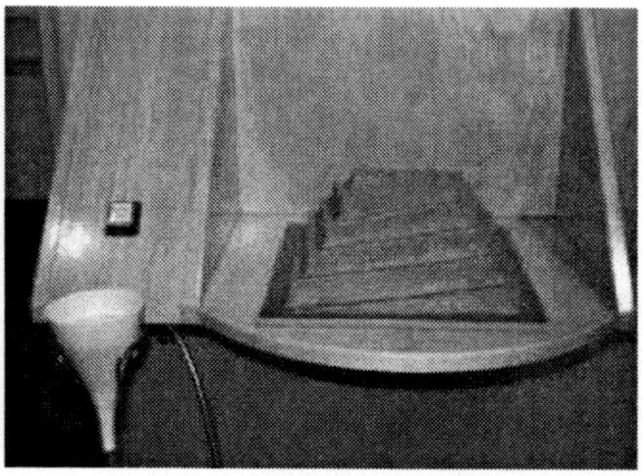

Figure 13 – Handheld audio device integrated into exhibit at Museum of Science Boston

the majority of positive comments were readability of video signs (n=7) and docents (n=11). Readability included issues related to “other” (overall readability) (n=4) and font size and style (n=3). The docent category consisted of comments about docents providing personal assistance for touching (“other”) (n=4), docents’ overall helpfulness and attitude (“other”) (n=4), sound of docents (n=2), and information sufficiency (n=2).

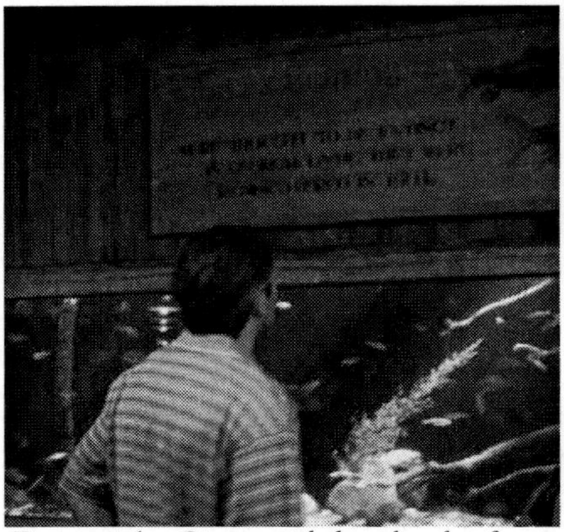

Figure 14 – Signs with low levels of lighting and low contrast at Redhorse Sucker Fish at the Georgia Aquarium.

Discussion

The findings from this study indicate that there are several characteristics that can be barriers or facilitators to accessing exhibits at the Georgia Aquarium: 1) display, including viewing height, interaction height, and visibility; 2) interpretation, including position, readability, lighting,

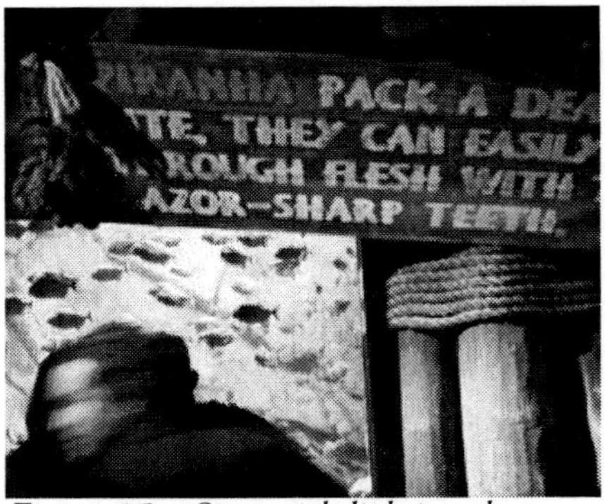

Figure 15 – Sign with lighting that casts shadows on text at Piranhas exhibit at the Georgia Aquarium.

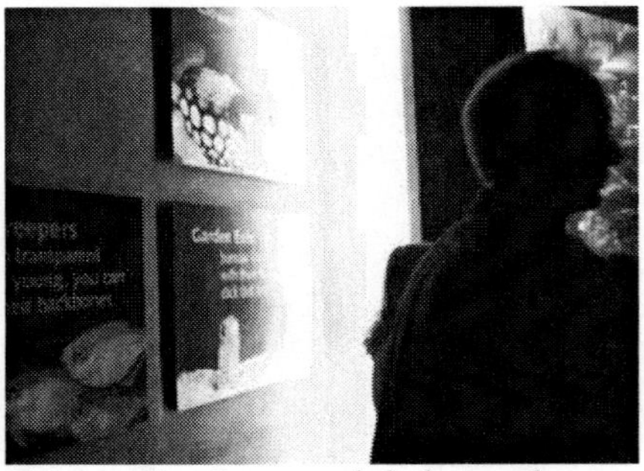

Figure 16 – Signs with lighting glare at Garden Eels and Glassy Sweepers exhibit at the Georgia Aquarium.

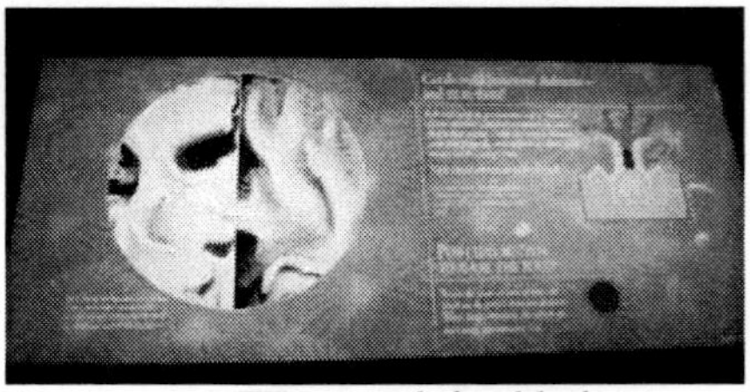

Figure 17 – Signs with backlighting at the Shedd Aquarium.

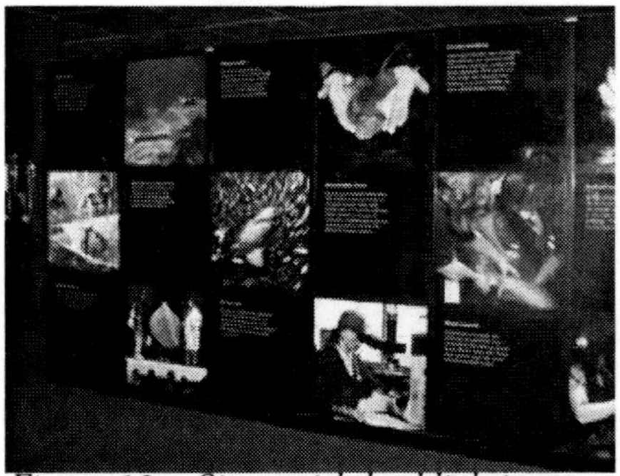

Figure 18 – Signs with backlighting at the National Aquarium in Baltimore.

visibility, and sufficiency; and 3) surrounding environment, including crowd and lighting.

Display. Viewing Height of Display. Viewing height of display was a barrier for individuals with motor impairments at a number of exhibits. Specifically, some touch tank walls, waterlines, and terrestrial floors were too high or too low, making it impossible for individuals who were seated (e.g., motor impairments) to view the animals. Additionally, immersion tunnels and domes were too low or short for individuals using wheelchairs to access. Conversely, individuals reported that several of the full wall exhibits (Figure 1) provided "good sight lines" and overhead tanks enabled them to "see past the crowd."

When viewing height of the display is too high or too low, possible solutions may include bringing the person up to a higher or lower level (e.g., ramp), providing an alternate viewing method (e.g., cameras, mirrors), and raising or lowering the display or a component of the display (e.g., waterline). Other institutions have dealt with similar issues related to viewing height of the display by having portals or small windows built into the display or creating an elevated area on the side of the display (Figure 2).

Interaction Height of Display. Interaction height of the display was also a problem for some of the participants at all of the touch tanks as a result of the display wall being too high for individuals to reach the animals. One way that the Aquarium has tried to make the touch tanks accessible is by using portable baskets. Interaction height barriers can also be accommodated through other techniques such as tanks that are shorter as in Figure 3, or narrower and shallower as shown in Figure 4.

Visibility of Display. Individuals with vision impairments

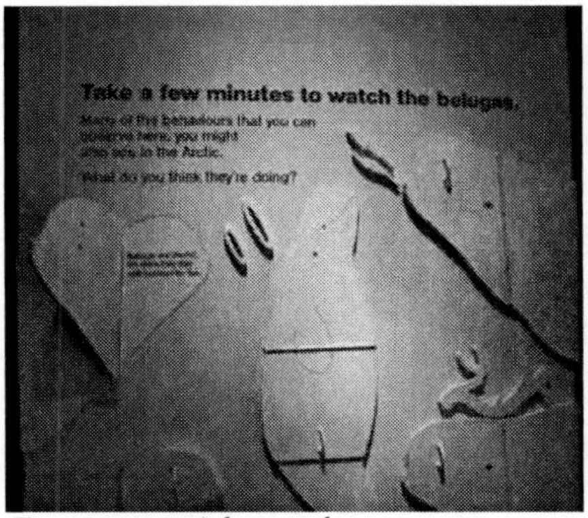

Figure 19 – A low-tech interactive sign at the Vancouver Aquarium

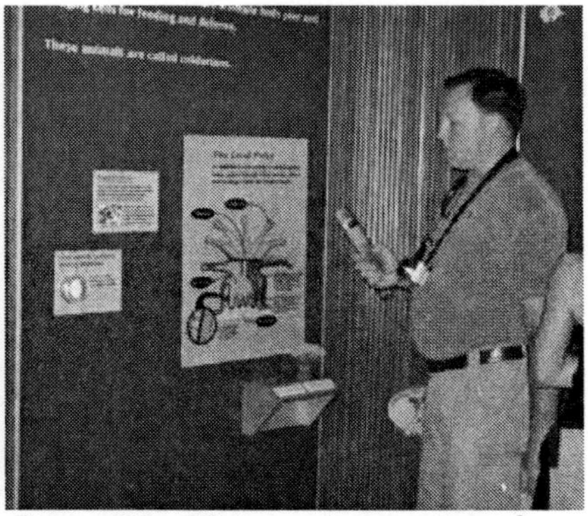

Figure 20 – Visitor using a personal audio tour at the Waikiki Aquarium.

indicated that they had difficulty seeing or knowing which animals were in the display. Docents were available in some of the larger exhibits and found to be helpful for individuals with vision impairments, especially when they provided detailed or comparative statements (e.g., the rays look like slow moving birds as they glide through the water) about the animals.

There are multiple ways of describing the animal that is in the display, including interpretation that is presented in signs or brochures, and in some cases, audio format (which will be discussed below in the Interpretation section). However, some individuals with vision impairments prefer to learn through touch. Some institutions have tactile representations of animals for visitors to interact with, including simulated (Figure 5) or real parts of animals (Figure 6), and scale models (Figure 7).

Position of Static Interpretation. Participants from all impairment groups, except cognitive, noted that in every gallery there were problems with interpretation that was too high and/or too far from the display. Specific examples included Cold Water Quest (i.e., Japanese Spider Crabs: too high, Beluga Whales: too far from display), Ocean Voyager (i.e., acrylic display: too high), and River Scout (i.e., Electric Fish: too high). It is worth mentioning that individuals who use wheelchairs were able to see the kiosks in the Tropical Diver Coral Reef and Georgia Explorer because they are mounted at a shorter height and angle.

Positioning interpretation for optimal access can provide a more educational experience. Some ways to do this are placing signs closer to displays (Figure 8), lowering signs (Figure 9), and providing alternative or personal solutions (e.g., audio tours, pamphlets).

Readability of Static Interpretation. The font size, style, or contrast on signs and kiosks in at least eight exhibits made it difficult for some individuals to read information (Figure 10). Individuals had problems with exhibits such as the printed signs near the first view of the River Otters in the Cold Water Quest (blends in), the kiosks in the Tropical Diver Coral Reef (font size too small), and the projected signs in the Tropical Diver Jellies (too fast and poor contrast) (Figure 11). Good examples of signage that were preferred by individuals were the video panel signs in the River Scout Arawana/Arapaima area (see Figure 12) and in the Tropical Diver Coral Reef.

Readability of signs and kiosks can be improved by increasing the font size, boldness and contrast, slowing down the speed of signs that change, and providing alternate formats. Some institutions have included an auditory component (Figure 13) or made the settings changes available to the user.

Lighting. Lighting to illuminate interpretation is closely tied to readability, but has its own impact on visual access. Lighting barriers can present as unevenness or shading, dimness (too dark), and glare. Participants noted that some signs were too dark, such as in Cold Water Quest (i.e., Japanese Spider Crabs, Sea Otters), River Scout (i.e., across from "crawl through"), and Georgia Explorer (i.e., Redhorse Sucker Fish) (Figure 14). Additionally, some signs had uneven or partially shaded lighting, as represented in Figure 15 at the River Scout Piranha exhibit, and some signs had a lot of glare, such as the Tropical Diver Garden Eels sign (Figure 16).

Interpretation that has associated lighting barriers can be made more accessible by providing unobstructed soft lighting that covers the entire surface and using non-reflective text surfaces. Some institutions use backlighting in signs to ensure better viewing from multiple angles (Figures 17, 18).

Visibility. When individuals experienced barriers related to visibility of interpretation, this indicated that they were not able to see or know what was on the sign or kiosk. For example, participants had difficulty with the Ocean Voyager Touch Panel and the Tropical Diver Coral Reef kiosks due to not knowing that they were touch-activated interpretation sources and not being able to see the information on the screens. In fact, comments included "[I] wouldn't know it was there" or "[I] wouldn't get anything out of it." Additionally, several comments were made about being able to find docents, as they typically either broadcast their voices over a speaker system, which make them hard to locate for asking one-on-one questions, or passively waited for individuals to approach them. Improving visibility of interpretation sources can be accomplished through strategies such as consistently positioning interpretation sources and informing visitors about these locations as well as including multi-sensory feedback or alternative access to information sources.

Information Sufficiency. Availability and quantity of interpretation was a barrier for individuals from almost all of the impairment groups. In some cases, participants wanted to know more about the animals than was available on signs (e.g., where they live, what they eat) and, in others, participants wanted to have information on each animal in the display. For example, several signs in River Scout only provided the name of the fish and the Tropical Diver Coral Reef kiosks had fish listed that could not be found in the tank and fish in the tank that could not be found on the kiosk.

Additional interpretation can be provided in a variety of formats and strategies including audio tours, accessible menu-driven systems on kiosks, or pamphlets. A current trend is to provide layered interpretation that provides a range of information from less detailed to more in-depth information. This can be incorporated into stand-alone interactives or personal systems and may be a low-tech sign that is placed near the exhibit (Figure 19) or high-tech electronic devices that are carried around (Figure 20).

Surrounding Physical Environment

Crowd. The popularity of the Georgia Aquarium can be evidenced by having over two million visitors before the first year anniversary. Participants with vision, motor, speech, and cognitive impairments noted challenges due to crowd sound, navigation, and viewing issues Individuals with vision impairments noted the greatest number of problems with the crowd.

The Aquarium did lower the number of visitors allowed in the galleries at one time. This improved the experience for visitors, but did not solve the problem. A solution would be to advertise to visitors with disabilities that there are days or times during the day when fewer people are expected. Additionally, some of the previously mentioned suggestions for providing alternative viewing or interaction experiences may be beneficial.

Lighting. From the entrance through many of the galleries, the Georgia Aquarium had many areas with very low levels of brightness. Additionally, the walls, floors, and ceilings were often the same dark color, and there were few navigational cues for visitors with vision impairments. Problems were mentioned in exhibits at the Ocean Voyager gallery, including the large viewing window, and Tropical Diver gallery, including the Garden Eels.

Lighting issues can be improved by changing the type and quantity of light, as well as the color and texture of the surfaces it shines on. A solution could be to install path lighting where the wall and floor meet similar to the lights installed in aisles of airplanes or movie theaters.

Summary

As mentioned in the introduction, this report informs on the effectiveness of current exhibit design practices at the Georgia Aquarium. It is our intention that the results of this study will provide documented evidence about the experiences of individuals with disabilities who visited the exhibits at the Georgia Aquarium.

It must be noted that there are a few key limitations of this study. The first is that the study recruited a small sample of participants. The sample was selected to include key constituents who could provide input on the exhibit design practices at the Georgia Aquarium. The study results were not intended to be generalizable to all people with similar disabilities, but to provide preliminary data on how specific functional limitations can affect the usability of certain exhibit features and characteristics.

Secondly, individuals with hearing impairments experienced exhibits with sign language interpreters who were hired by the investigators for the purpose of the study. This created a situation where it is likely that fewer barriers were reported by these individuals. As this was the only means for participants with hearing impairments to understand what was said by the docents, as well as by other visitors during question and answer periods, it is suggested that the Aquarium explore contracting with an interpreter services.

Finally, the study was a broad review, not an in-depth analysis. These results are intended to not only create an awareness of usability problems, but to inform Aquarium staff and other interested investigators on future research directions. The Aquarium is a state-of-the-art facility that generally represents current design practice in the field of ILEs. However, as we experienced in this study, even the most well-intended designs may not be usable by all individuals. Usability testing that incorporates users with varying abilities throughout the design process typically leads to better outcomes. Additionally, future studies should analyze and test key characteristics of current and potential exhibits, before costly or significant changes are implemented. Moreover, a more inclusive and rigorous approach will support the development of future research objectives and ideally, change design practices by incorporating the needs of individuals with disabilities—leading to more universally designed exhibits.

References

[1] US Access Board, Americans with Disabilities Act Accessibility Guidelines, Department of Justice, Editor. 2004, Federal Register.

[2] Czaja, S., Hand Anthropometrics. 1984, Technical paper prepared for the U.S. Architectural and Transportation Barriers Compliance Board: Washington, DC.

[3] Jones, M.L. and J.A. Sanford, People with mobility impairments in the United States today and in 2010. Assistive Technology, 1996. 8(1): p. 43-52.

[4] Museum of Science Boston. Universal Design (Accessibility): Considerations for Designers. 2001 [cited May 20, 2005]; Available from: http://www.mos.org/exhibitdevelopment/access/design.html.

[5] Smithsonian Institution Press, Smithsonian Guidelines for Accessible Exhibition Design. 1996, Washington, D.C.: Smithsonian Institution Press.

[6] National Endowment for the Arts, Design for Accessibility: A Cultural Administrator's Handbook. 2003, Washington, D.C.

[7] Salmen, J., Everyone's Welcome: The Americans with Disabilities Act and Museums. 1998, Washington, D.C.: American Association of Museums Bookstore.

Aging, Disability and Independence
W.C. Mann (Ed.)
IOS Press, 2008

doi:10.3233/978-1-58603-902-8-57

An Integrated Structure of Intelligent Techniques for Enhancing Easy Controllability of Service Robots

Hyong-Euk Lee[1], Jun-Hyeong Do[2], Yong-Hwi Kim[2], Heon-Hui Kim[1], Kwang-Hyun Park[2], and Z. Zenn Bien[2]
[1]Human-friendly Welfare Robot System Engineering Research Center, KAIST,
373-1 Guseong-Dong, Yuseong-Gu, Daejeon 305-701, KOREA
[2]Department of Electrical Engineering and Computer Science, KAIST
373-1 Guseong-Dong, Yuseong-Gu, Daejeon 305-701, KOREA

Abstract: In this paper, we propose an integrated structure of intelligent techniques to enhance easy-controllability of service robots for the elderly and people with disabilities in a smart home environment. Intelligent techniques have been implemented in human-robot interfaces according to the 3 categories of intelligence, toward enhancing controllability. First, a gesture-recognition system has been implemented toward a more intuitive/natural human-robot interface. Second, a task planning system plays a role to simplify possible commands by the user to control various kinds of devices/ robotic agents, for given well-structured tasks. Third, we applied a life-long learning system for intention reading of the user to provide service tasks automatically in advance of his/her explicit command instruction.

I. Introduction

Today, many countries confront the demographic shift toward an aging population. As a result, the portion of people, who need assistance in daily life activities, is increasing faster than the availability of caregivers. Note that many industrial systems have successfully replaced human labor with autonomous systems. These systems work efficiently and with performance improvement while eliminating tedious, difficult, and dangerous jobs for people. It may also be possible to address the shortage of human caregivers withs 'robot caregivers' using technological solutions such as IT and robotics.

In the area of service robotics, various robotic systems have been developed to help people in the home environment and public places. Robots that perform work and tasks for people are called service robots [1]. Service tasks, for example, include fetching and delivering items, including food, as well as rendering entertainment services such as control of appliances [2][3][4]. In larger environments, such as office buildings, hospitals, or museums, service robots could provide guiding services as well as delivering items [5][6][7].

Rehabilitation robots are specialized service robots designed to assist people with disabilities. For example, KARES II [3] was designed to assist with daily life tasks for people with the spinal cord injury. Using various human-machine interfaces, KARES II performs 12 predefined service tasks, such as assisting with drinking and eating, turning a switch on/off, and picking up objects. FRIEND [8] and Care-O-Bot II [9] also assist people with disabilities in daily activities.

For the design of a service robot, Leifer [10] proposed three rules: (1) service robots should be designed as social agents; (2) service robots have to tolerate ambiguity; (3) all applications should be reapplications. The objective of this design philosophy is to develop service robots as social agents that can interact with humans in a friendly way. The robot should have proper human-like intelligence to be aware of what to do, where to go, and so on, even when it is not told precisely about the detailed actions to achieve a given task. Leifer also asserts that the system applications should be implemented with proven technologies and assured confidence for success because with humans involved, trial-and-error is not acceptable.

Different than with general-purpose service robots, in designing an assistive service robot, characteristics of the target user must be analyzed first, and then, the required service tasks and design specifications are based on this analysis. Specifically, when we consider the elderly and/or people with disabilities as target users, an additional aspect to be considered is that they may have difficulty in controlling complex robotic systems and in reacting rapidly to unexpected situations. Service tasks should be performed autonomously with ease by the robot's own intelligence for the given task command.

In this paper we discuss the intelligent techniques which can be utilized for a service robot. We consider a steward robot, which can provide service tasks for the inhabitant of a smart house. In this situation, human beings, controllable devices, and robotic agents are considered as subsystems in a large-scale system.

Note that the available number of services increases as the number of controllable devices and service agents increases.

However, it is quite difficult to control all the target devices, especially for older people and people with disabilities. Therefore, we focus on the intelligent techniques for enhancing easy-controllability.

This paper is organized as follows. In the next section we briefly describe the types of intelligence considered essential to enhance easy-controllability in a service-robot integrated smart house. Following this, we discuss an integrated structure of intelligent techniques within our smart house environment, called Intelligent Sweet Home (ISH), and its components including the steward robot Joy. Next we explain the detailed systems with intelligent techniques: 1) a gesture recognition system, 2) a task planning system, and 3) a life-long learning system. We end with brief concluding remarks.

Concept of Intelligence for Enhancing Controllability in a Service-Robot Integrated Environment

The words 'intelligence' and 'intelligent system' have been widely used. However, it seems they are used differently from one system to another [11]. Albus insisted that a useful definition of intelligence should span a wide range of capabilities, from those well understood to those beyond comprehension, include both biological and machine embodiments, and span an intellectual range from an insect to Einstein, from a thermostat to the most sophisticated computer system that could ever be built [12]. Also, since the notion of "intelligent control" was first proposed by Fu [13] as human-like control in automation, various intelligent methodologies have been introduced to increase the flexibility and range of the mathematical model-based automatic control system. Also, the concept of intelligence has been extended with the aid of artificial intelligence, including fuzzy logic, neural networks, evolutionary computation, and approximate reasoning techniques [11]. These techniques are sometimes utilized in a single form or in a hybrid form to fulfill the performance objectives of the target system [2].

However, general notions on intelligence do not provide any specified guidelines to design a practical system because the required type of intelligence varies according to the target application. For example, intelligence on knowledge abstraction and information fusion is important in the financial/economic analysis field while cognitive intelligence is more important in the biometrics field. Also, intelligence on accurate manipulation/ control in uncertain environments is required more in the robotics area.

Recall that we focus on the aspect of easy-controllability. In general, the interaction between two agents occurs throughout one or more interfaces. In the industrial field, the interfaces are simple, specialized tools such as buttons, and joysticks. For human-computer interaction, keyboard/mouse, a joysticks, touch pads have been utilized. Also, various forms of graphic user interfaces have also been paralleled with the conventional interfaces, emphasizing the aspect of visualization.

However, the question of how to use conventional interfaces becomes more complex as the number of available control functions increases. An engineering solution to handle this difficulty may be a more intuitive/natural method of control command by intelligent techniques. Observe that human intention can be expressed in various forms such as voice, gestures, facial expressions. If a human-robot interface can recognize human intention from such features by means of intelligent techniques, it will be a more intuitive and convenient interface in a human-centered system, compared with artificially made interfaces. We may call it the first level of intelligence. We will further show a gesture recognition system as a successful example in a later section of this paper.

Even though we have appropriate interfaces, it is still cumbersome to give control commands for varying situations, especially in a complex environment with robotic agents. Therefore we introduce the second level of intelligence which provides a higher level of autonomy. Note that some tasks may require more than one subsystem for cooperative execution. For example, we have to consider the aspect of possible collision when we control two or more mobile robots simultaneously. In this case, if higher level of intelligence is available, the robot can generate a sequence of subtasks, distribute subtasks to subsystems, and supervise actions of each subsystem to synchronize the subtask. This reduces the cognitive load of the human operator. Task planning [18] is a good example of implementing this kind of intelligence for enhancing task execution efficiency. By simplifying possible commands by the user, the user can control the target system more easily as he/she intended.

The third level of intelligence is an extension of the second level, which aims 'disappearing commands' from 'simplifying commands' by means of learning capability. If a robot can recognize human intention such as behavioral preference, the robot can provide service tasks in advance of the user's explicit command instruction. This kind of robot can be called an 'active service robot,' rather than a 'passive service robot' which provides service tasks only for the given command as conventional service robots. When a system recognizes human bio-signals and behavior in the short term, with an assumption that selected features of the target pattern remain stationary, a typical classifier is quite successful in performance, especially with various soft-computing techniques employed in the process of perception and recognition [19]. If the system must operate in a residential service environment for a long period of time, however, such an approach may not work because we must deal with time-varying and non-stationary learning targets, e.g. human behavioral pattern/preference, for a long time span. As such, the learning capability becomes an important factor to address such data patterns in view of long term learning and adaptation for human-friendly interaction.

These 3 types of intelligence are summarized in Fig. 1. Further, we shall show successful examples of implementing intelligent techniques in a layered structure in the next section.

A Layered Structure of Intelligent Techniques in Intelligent Sweet Home and Steward Robot Joy

As a practical application platform, we introduce a smart house environment which has been developed at KAIST. The Intelligent Sweet Home (ISH) allows people with movement limitations to perform various complicated everyday tasks independently in a residential space [14]. Based on the results of a questionnaire

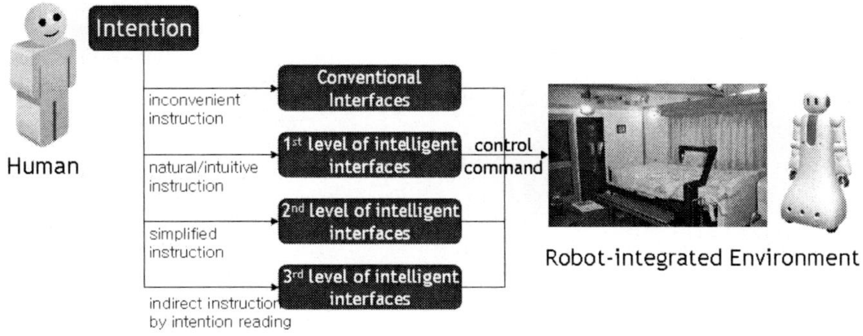

Fig. 1. The types of intelligent interfaces in view of easy-controllability

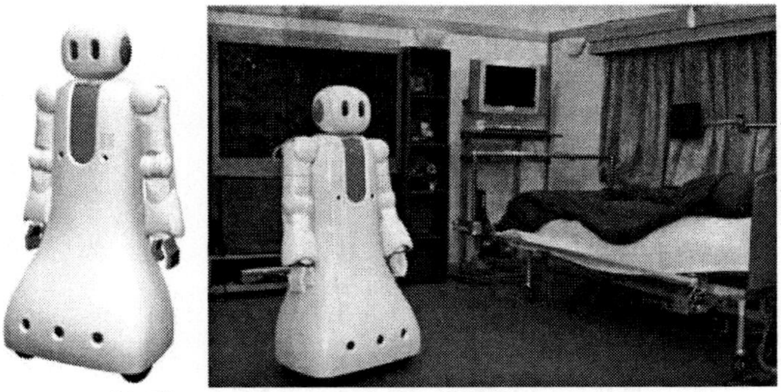

Fig. 2. Steward robot Joy in Intelligent Sweet Home

survey [15], we designed the ISH to provide the services residents need, such as independence in going outdoors, assistance in meal preparation, eating, drinking, control of home appliances from the bed or wheelchair, and bringing/removing objects while in the bed.

The ISH includes several robotic modules such as an intelligent bed, intelligent wheelchair and robotic hoist to assist motion and mobility, and human-machine interaction modules to provide a natural and convenient means of transferring information between the user and the devices installed in the home. All home-installed components are connected via a home network that includes both wired and wireless communication modules. Referring to the user's commands, the central unit

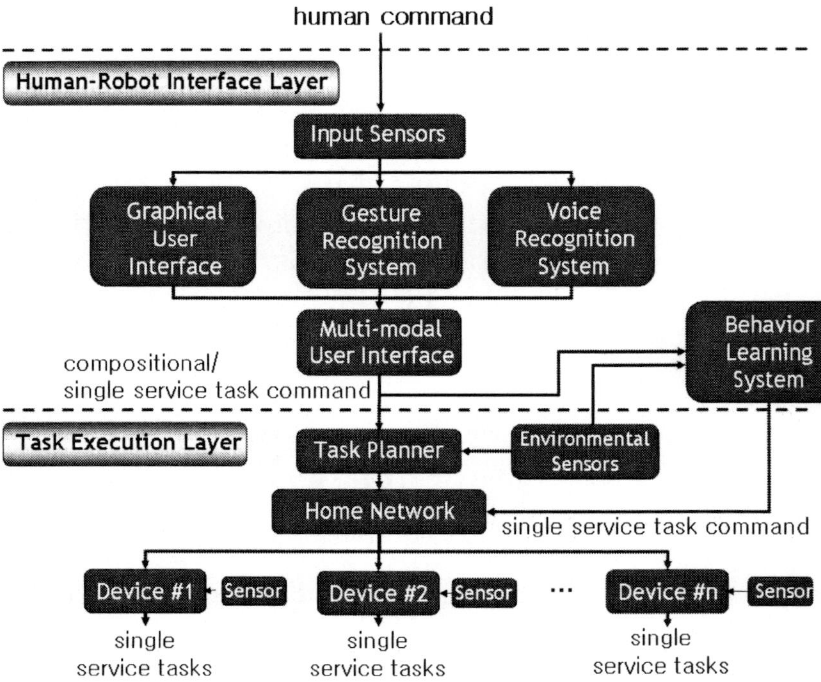

Fig. 3. An integrated software structure of the ISH and the Steward Robot Joy

generates a set of actions for each agent and the sequence in which these actions will be executed. Most of the assistive modules developed have been designed to perform their inherent functions as well as to cooperate in tasks with other related systems.

Since the ISH consists of a number of subsystems and tasks, and each task requires usually more than one subsystem for cooperative execution, the user has to control and command all the subsystems by various corresponding human-machine interfaces. To resolve this difficulty, we have developed a steward robot, named Joy, as shown in Fig. 2 so that the user can operate the whole system easily [21]. One of the key features of the steward robot is learning capability, including intention reading so that some awkward or difficult situations can be avoided for the user with physical disabilities. The system is also supposed to provide a personalized service depending on the resident's preference and life style. All of these functions of the robot will enable the home system to perform appropriate tasks autonomously by observing the resident's behavior instead of with cumbersome manual operations.

We described the 3 types of intelligent interfaces to enhance easy-controllability in the previous section. Based on this approach, we have developed an integrated software/hardware structure of intelligent techniques as shown in Fig. 3. In view of multi-modality, various types of human commands can be handled by the human-robot interfaces. Also, the task planning system can generate appropriate sequence of decomposed tasks from the given compositional task command. Further, the behavior learning system can recommend the desired control commands based on the acquired behavior patterns of an inhabitant. Each of the systems has been realized with appropriate

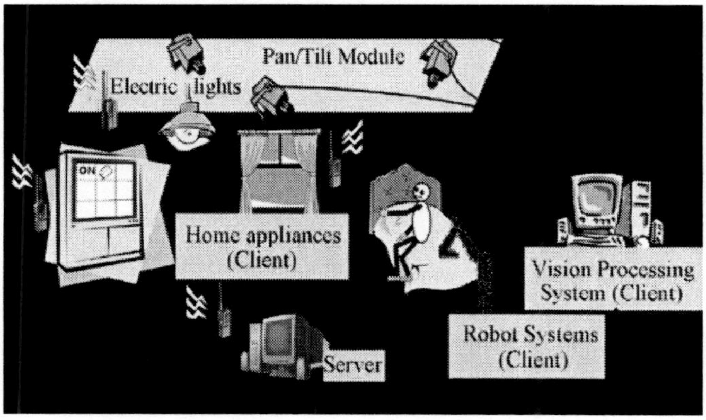

Fig. 4. Soft remote control system in the Intelligent Sweet Home

intelligent techniques, which are further explained in the next section.

Intelligent Techniques in the Layered Structure

The Gesture-Recognition System

First, we explain a human-machine interface, called "soft remote control system", which is a hand gesture recognition-based interface. The soft remote control system allows the user to control various home appliances naturally in a smart house without body-attached devices [16]. Fig. 4 shows the overall configuration of the soft remote control system. Multiple color cameras with a pan/tilt/zoom module are used to acquire the images of the room. In the vision processing system, the user's hand gesture commands are analyzed and the information about them is transferred to the home server via TCP/IP. Then, the home server sends Infrared (IR) signals to control the home appliances.

The command procedure to operate a function of a specific device is defined in a simple and natural way that the user can command easily and intuitively. The user first selects the device he/she wants to control by pointing to it. Then, the user can command the operation of desired functions via 10 predefined basic hand motion commands which consist of 1-D motion and 2-D motion. If there is no command gesture in a few seconds, the activated device is released. Otherwise, the user can command other functions to the currently activated device. To address errors in recognizing the user's pointing directions, we developed the concept of feedback by which the user can adjust the pointing direction and confirm the recognition result.

In case the pointing direction is beside the target, the soft remote control system finds the closest appliance to the current pointing direction, and announces to the user which direction his/her pointing hand should be moved to adjust the pointing direction by displaying the location of the target and currently pointed spot. The display also shows the selected device and recognized command gesture when a device is pointed at, and an operation of the selected device is commanded, respectively, by the user.

When the user commands by hand gestures through the soft remote control system, ordinary gestures may seem to be similar to the predefined command gestures. This results in a recognition error because those similar gestures could be recognized as commands by the system. To resolve this problem, fuzzy garbage model has been proposed [17].

The fuzzy garbage model is a fuzzy model defined by meaningless but similar gestures to commands. Those gestures are called garbage in this paper. Also, a fuzzy command model is defined by the command gestures. Each model is constructed by the corresponding fuzzy rules and membership functions, and produces the output score, which indicates that the input gesture belongs to each class. By comparing the output score, the user's gesture is recognized as a garbage or command.

The Task-Planning System

In the ISH, service tasks are categorized as follows [22]: 1) low-level task: the task required to control a single target device (i.e., turning on/off the TV) and 2) high-level task: the task required to control multiple target devices with a proper sequence (i.e., preparing to go out, preparing a meal). For example, a person with lower-limb paralysis wants to get out of bed in the ISH. In this case, the target person, who has mobility impairment, has to control the intelligent bed robot, the robotic hoist, the intelligent wheelchair, the steward robot Joy, and the other devices in a proper sequence to reduce task performance time and to avoid possible collisions between the mobile agents. Recall that this process requires cumbersome manual operations, and it is quite difficult for people with disabilities to conduct such operations under possibly unexpected situations.

Therefore, to resolve this difficulty, a task planning system was proposed for the steward robot Joy to control subsystems automatically in a proper sequence. Based on the observation of the environmental status and the device status, the task planning system generates an appropriate sequence of low-level tasks from the given high-level task.

Task planning means, in general, the capability to find a sequence from an initial state to a goal state in a way that all facts of the goal state are true. Here, a fact denotes for the discrete status of a device and a state is a set of the facts. The goal state is given by a high-level task and the initial state is decided by environmental sensory information.

We present a task planning system based on the STRIPS (STanford Research Institute Problem Solver) representation [23]

[24]. Until now, many task planning systems have been developed under the STRIPS representation such as Graphplan [25], BSR-Graphplan [26], and Split planning [27]. Among them, we found that the split planning method showed better performance than the other planning algorithms in view of computation time as long as under the condition that the number of facts in an initial state is larger than that in a goal state [22].

However, the computation time is still too large to be applied in a practical system. To handle this problem, we applied a backward graph construction scheme to the existing split planning with a state partitioning technique. Fig. 5 shows the overall structure of the proposed task planning system.

As shown in Fig. 5, the task planning system consists of four kinds of the processing modules: an initial planning module, a state partitioning module, BSP (Backward Split Planning) modules, and a sequence merging module. For the given high-level task and the observed sensory information, the initial planning module generates an initially planned graph based on the STRIPS representation. Then, the initial graph is decomposed into a collection of several sub-problems in the state partitioning module. For each sub-problem, the BSP module generates the planning result, which is a sequence of actions. Finally, each sequence is merged into a sequence of actions for the original problem.

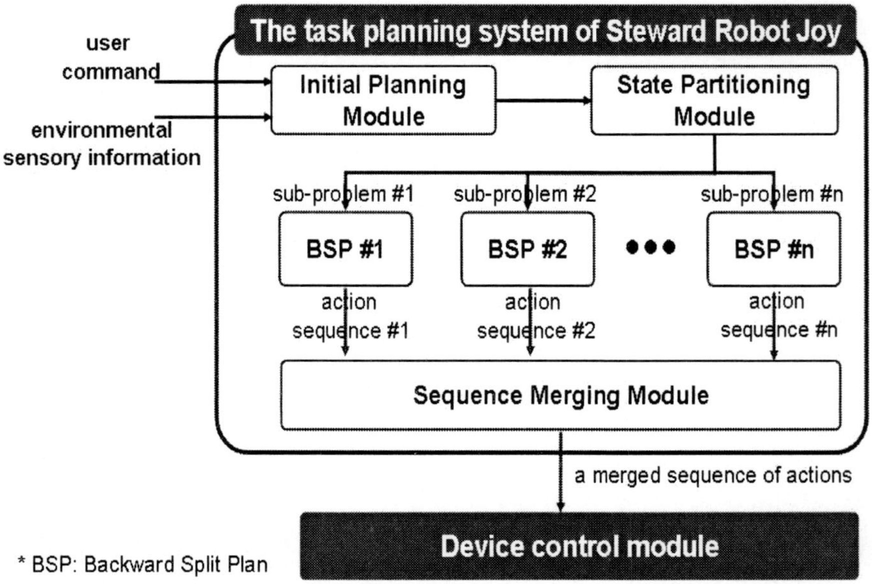

Fig. 5. Overall structure of the task planning system

Behavior Pattern Learning System

Finally, we present a probabilistic fuzzy rule-based learning system for intention reading based on behavioral pattern of the inhabitant in the ISH in view of realizing the third level of intelligence. Recall that the user can express his/her intention directly to the target machine using the human-machine interface. It is an effective and accurate way to control target devices. However, sometimes it may also be inconvenient because the user has to be involved in their control loops frequently. The learning system, on the other hand, reads the user's intention with an indirect method, for example, by observing his/her behavioral patterns. It allows the robot to provide its available service intelligently in advance of the user's direct command.

The learning system is a subcomponent of the steward robot Joy, as shown in Fig. 2, which is applied for learning the resident's behavioral patterns. The learning system collects behavioral patterns of the resident according to the available sensory information, converts in an appropriate knowledge form, and utilizes the acquired knowledge to control target devices.

In general, an appropriate learning model and a learning algorithm are selected based on analysis about their learning target. In most pattern classification/learning problems, data patterns with well-separable classes are considered as the learning target. However, the human behavioral pattern and some physiological bio-signals (e.g., EEG, EMG, ECG, etc.) show complex characteristics such as high dimensionality, nonlinear-coupling of attributes, subjectivity, apparent inconsistency, susceptibility to environments and disturbances, and time-variance as well as situation-dependency [2], and therefore, it is

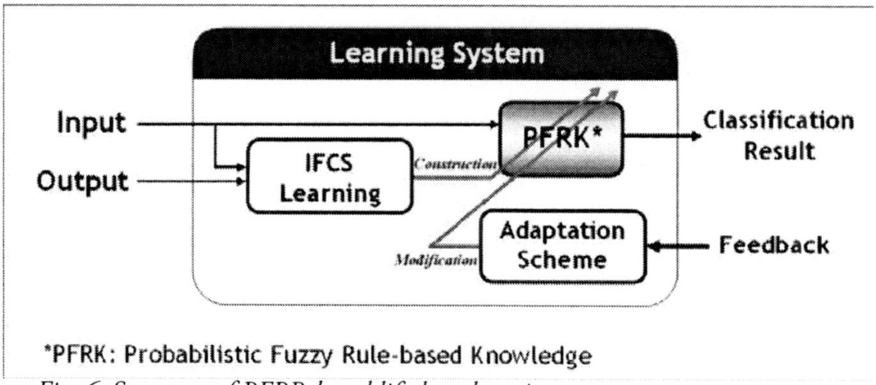

Fig. 6. Structure of PFRB-based life-long learning system

difficult to handle them with a complete mathematical model.

Note that in practical situations, possible measurement data by available sensors are limited for behavioral pattern monitoring, and thus I/O training examples can be sparse and may contain apparently inconsistent examples. Therefore, we select PFRB (probabilistic fuzzy rule base) as a knowledge representation type to handle such inconsistent characteristics of the target data pattern. Also, we have proposed IFCS (Iterative Fuzzy Clustering with Supervision) algorithm to extract meaningful PFRB from numerical data patterns [20]. Furthermore, to handle time-varying characteristics of the target data pattern, a life-long learning structure with an adaptation scheme based on the four interconnected functional memory blocks, which are STM (Short-Term Memory), ITM (Interim-Transition Memory), LTM (Long-term Memory), and ABM (Action-Buffer Memory). Fig. 6 shows the overall learning architecture of the proposed learning system.

The proposed learning system can be utilized to a home appliance control system in the ISH. For example, the learning system has been used as a TV viewing genre/channel recommendation system. The learning system can recommend the resident's favorite TV genre/channel based on the acquired probabilistic fuzzy rule-based knowledge in sequential order.

V. Concluding Remarks

In this paper, we have presented an integrated structure of intelligent techniques for enhancing easy-controllability perspective in a service robot-integrated smart house environment. The intelligent techniques have been utilized in a single/hybridized form in the layered structure. The proposed system is thought to be helpful especially for the elderly and people with disabilities so that the system reduces the cognitive load of the users as well as possible complicated commands. Note that machine intelligence is currently an active research area toward human intelligence. It includes not only logical contents but also physical contents, and emotional contents. To realize/implement a desired functional intelligence, we finally remark that various kinds of hybridizing/modifying the existing intelligent techniques are still available and their methodologies are thought to be challenging issues.

Acknowledgement
This work was supported by the SRC/ERC program of the MOST/KOSEF under grant #R11-1999-008.

References

[1] Hillman, M. (2003). Rehabilitation robotics from past to present-historical perspective, in Proceedings of International Conference on Rehabilitation Robots 2003, Daejeon, Korea.

[2] Bien, Z., & Lee, H.-E. (2007). Effective Learning System Techniques for Human-Robot Interaction in Service Environment, Knowledge-based Systems, 20(5), 439-456.

[3] Bien, Z., Park, K. H., Kim, D. J., & Jung, J. W. (2004). Welfare-oriented service robotic systems: Intelligent Sweet Home & KARES II, Lecture Notes in Control and Information Sciences, 306, 57-94.

[4] Balaguer, C., Gimenez, A., Huete, A., Sabatini, A., Topping, M., & Bolmsjo, G. (2006). The MATS robot: service climbing robot for personal assistance, Robotics & Automation Magazine, IEEE, 13(1), 32-41.

[5] Hada, Y., & Takase, K. (2004). Delivery service robot using distributed acquisition, actuators and intelligence, Proceedings of the 2004 IEEE/RSJ International Conference on Intelligent Robots and Systems.

[6] Bandini, S., & Manzoni, S. (2004). Experience with CiceRobot, a museum guide cognitive robot, Lecture notes in computer science, 3673, 474-482.

[7] Bischoff, R., & Graefe, V. (2004). HERMES-A versatile personal robotic assistant, Proceedng of the IEEE, 92(11).

[8] Volosyak, I., Kouzmitcheva, O., Ristic, D., & Graser, A. (2005). Improvement of visual perceptual capabilities by feedback structures for robotic system FRIEND, IEEE Transactions on systems, man, and cybernetics-Part C: Applications and review, 35(1).

[9] Graf, B., Hans, M., & Schraft, D. (2004). Care-O-bot II-Development of a next generation robotic home assistant, Autonomous Robots, 16, 193-205.

[10] Leifer, L. (1995). Tele-service Robots: integrating the socio-technical Framework of Human Service through the Internet-WWW, in Proceedings of International Workshop on Biorobotics: Human-Robot Symbiosys, Japan.

[11] Bien, Z., Bang, W.-C., Kim, D.-Y., & Han, J.-S. (2002). Machine Intelligence Quotient: its measurements and applications, Fuzzy Set and Systems, 127, 3-16.

[12] Albus, J. S. (1991). Outline for a theory of intelligence, IEEE Transactions on System, Man, and Cybernetics, 21(3), 473-509.

[13] Fu, K. S. (1970). Learning control system-review and outlook, IEEE Transactions on Automatic Control, 10(5), 327-342.

[14] Bien, Z., Chang, P.-H., Yoon, Y.-S., Park, K.-H., Park, S.H., Park, S., et al. (2007). Realization and Evaluation of Assistive Human-Mechatronic Systems with Human-friendly Robotic Agents at HWRS-ERC, Proc. of the 2007 IEEE Int'l Conf. on Rehabilitation Robotics, 328-334.

[15] Kim, Y., Park, K.-H., Seo, K.-H., Kim, C. H., Lee, W.-J., Song, W.-G., et al. (2003). A report on questionnaire for developing Intelligent Sweet Home for the disabled and the elderly in Korean living conditions, Proc. of the 2003 Int'l Conf. on Rehabilitation Robotics, 171-174.

[16] Do, J.-H., Jung, S. H., Yang, S.-E., Jang, H., Jung, J.-W., & Bien, Z. (2007). Gesture-based Interface using Multiple Cameras for Home Appliance Control, International Journal of Assistive Robotics and Mechatronics, 8(2), 37-43.

[17] Yang, S.-E. (2007). Gesture Spotting using Fuzzy Garbage Model and User Adaptation, Master dissertation, School of Electrical Engineering & Computer Science, Division of Electrical Engineering, KAIST, Daejeon, Korea

[18] Valle, S. M. L. (2006). Planning algorithms, Cambridge University Press.

Aging, Disability and Independence
W.C. Mann (Ed.)
IOS Press, 2008

doi:10.3233/978-1-58603-902-8-71

It's all about the Information: The Role of Informatics in Telecare

A. P. Glascock[1], D. M. Kutzik[2]
[1,2] Drexel University, Department of Culture and Communication, Philadelphia, PA, USA

Abstract: As Telecare becomes increasingly a component of care models, there must be a shift away from the current emphasis on the technology used to collect and transfer data, toward a focus on the information provided to caregivers and the subsequent actions and outcomes. In response to this need, the Caring Home Initiative, a multi-year, multi-site study that collects evidence on the use of Telecare in real world care environments, was undertaken.

Researchers in each of six current Caring Home Sites are using a common set of instruments: 1) an intake protocol to collect comparable information on each of the clients; 2) the TAO (i.e., "trigger-action-outcome") web-based data entry system with alert, trend and query forms to record each time information provided by technology is used in care provision; 3) an interview schedule for the actual users of the system and, where possible, a family member of the user; and 4) a questionnaire given to formal caregivers.

The findings of the CHI show that: first the information provided by an integrated Telecare system is reliable, valid and most importantly, timely; second, automated, continuously updated, electronic wellbeing records can be generated by the imPACS (i.e., analytics and decision support) component of the system; and third, the integrated system can also automatically generate continuously updated care delivery records.

The main lesson learned from the CHI is that if the goal of Telecare is to produce a product for use by caregivers, then integration among the three levels—technology, care and informatics— is essential

Keywords: Behavioral Informatics, Telecare, home care, electronic records

Introduction

The vital role of informatics in the growth of Telecare has been largely underestimated because of the logical but unwarranted emphasis on the technology that is used to collect and transmit the data/information. While the authors have been instrumental in the development of some of this technology [5], over the last several years it has become evident that to fully realize Telecare's full potential, the multiple roles played by informatics must be better understood. In order for this to happen at least three changes in the way Telecare is viewed must take place. First, Telecare must be viewed as "essentially a service delivery innovation supported by new technology and existing technology used in new ways" [4] rather than as a clever technology that is going to transform health care. Second, Telecare is a care provision tool and, as such, it is only useful once it is integrated into an existing care model—it is not a care model itself. And finally, there has to be a much greater emphasis on the information that Telecare collects, transforms and transfers. In particular, there must be an increased emphasis on the collection of "data on the changing care outcomes, delivery processes (e.g. impact on jobs and work practices) and costs and savings as the scheme (Telecare) is being deployed and mainstreamed" [4].

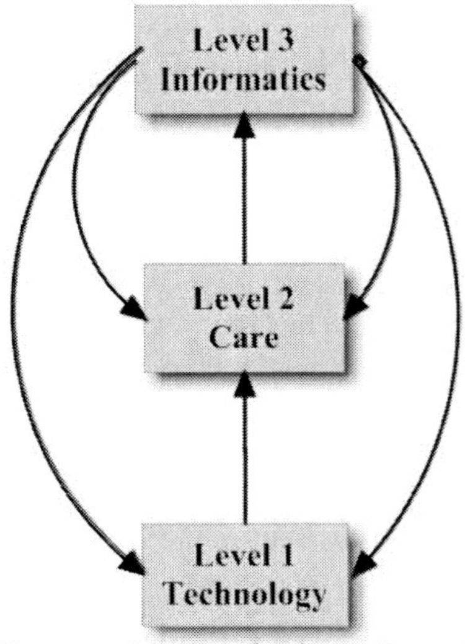

Figure 1: Integrated Telecare System

Objectives

The need for this last change in emphasis is what has driven the creation of the Caring Home Initiative (CHI), a multi-year, multi-site study that collects evidence on the use of Telecare in real world care environments. Except in a few cases [2] [3], most reports on the effectiveness of Telecare focus almost exclusively on case study/ anecdotes: how a life was saved, how care was altered for a particular client. These anecdotes are often compelling, but as a wise researcher once said, "anecdotes are not data". Thus, what is clearly needed to understand Telecare's effectiveness as a care provision tool is an evidentiary study that places emphasis on the information.

The CHI assumes that for Telecare to be effective, three different levels must be integrated into a comprehensive system: 1) the technology level which collects the data, translates it into information and transfers it to the next level; 2) the care level that receives the information and takes action; and 3) the informatics level that compiles the information from the other two levels into permanent records. Figure 1 depicts these three levels and suggests how they are interdependent. For example, without the Second Level to take action, the data produced by the technology in Level 1 have no real purpose and without the data produced by the technology, there is nothing to indicate that action needs to be taken at Level 2. Likewise, without a way to track and record the actions taken at Level 2, there is no means of evaluating the effectiveness of the actions on either the individual requiring the care or the care delivery model.

The remainder of this paper is a report of selected findings of the CHI to date, specifically focusing on how the three levels operate to provide an integrated system to be used in the delivery of care to older, frail individuals. The CHI began in late 2003 with the first installations of a commercialized version of a behavioral monitoring system, QuietCare™, and continues today with the study of three locations in England, four in the United States and one in the Netherlands. When the study is completed in 2009, it is anticipated that 14 locations in four countries with a total of 300-350 installations will have been studied. The analysis presented is both chronological and sequential and each level will be discussed separately. The discussion is divided into these three levels for ease of description and the levels are actually one and the same, as will be shown in the discussion section.

Methods

One of the major strengths of the ongoing CHI is that researchers in each of the locations use a common set of instruments: 1) an intake protocol to collect comparable information on each of the clients; 2) the TAO web-based alert, trend and query forms to record each time information provided by technology is used in care provision; 3) an interview schedule for the actual users of the system and, where possible, a family member of the user; and 4) a questionnaire to be given to formal caregivers. The key instrument is the TAO which stands for trigger, action and outcome and is filled out by the caregiver each time an alert is received, records the specific action taken by the caregiver and tracks the client's outcome in order to assess the effectiveness of the action.

The TAO provides the link between the alerts generated by the technology in Level 1, the care actions taken in Level 2 and the information products produced in Level 3. As such, the TAO is a diagnostic tool in that it continuously assesses the technology's reliability and validity. For example: are the thresholds used to generate alerts set at a meaningful level to reduce false alarms; was there an appropriate and timely response to a specific alert; can the tracking charts incorporated in the wellbeing record be used to improve care. Thus, the TAO's feedback loops, depicted in Figure 1, provide a self-correcting component at each of the three levels, while at the same time creating two types of electronic records: 1) a wellbeing record for the individual being monitored; and 2) a record of care delivery, including staff accountability and best practice.

Results

Level 1—The Technology

Although the main thrust of the CHI is on the informatics' level, it is necessary to briefly discuss the other two levels. The technology used in the QuietCare™ system is configured to collect data on: 1) wake up time; 2) meal preparation; 3) medication adherence; 4) overnight toileting; and 5) general activity. In addition, the system monitors the ambient temperature in the residence and provides "possible fall" notification. The data are translated into actionable information and displayed on a PIN secure web site that can be accessed by formal and/or informal caregivers. Both urgent and non-urgent alerts are sent, via email, text message and/or pager to caregivers, and information on both the client's activities and the action taken by caregivers is charted and displayed in a variety of tables and charts [5].

QuietCare's™ website presents the information on each activity into icons and clear narrative statements that relay the most important trends as simply as possible. Current day information is automatically compared to previously collected activity data to determine changes in activity. Green status indicators are displayed when the data show no significant deviation in the frequency and/or timing of data for a given activity; yellow status indicators are displayed when the frequency and timing of a given activity is higher or lower than expected; and red status indicators are displayed when a still higher threshold of deviation is recorded. Current day and historical information about the activities of the monitored individuals are displayed in various ways. The caregiver may look at a group summary page to get a quick sense of the status of a group of monitored individuals, or may drill

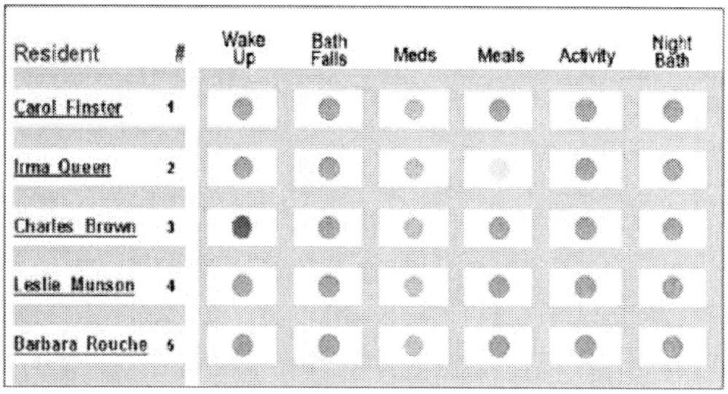

Figure 2: Institutional Summary Page

down to get very detailed information about the present or past activities of a given individual. Figure 2 is an example of a group event summary page of the kind used in a variety of institutional and homecare settings. The grayscale circles in this figure are the status indicators which appear as green, yellow or red on the actual website.

Red and yellow alerts are sent to the designated caregiver who initiates the TAO by clicking on the specified server and opening a "form" which is auto-populated with information about the client, the alert(s) in question and which asks the caregiver to check boxes and fill in text fields relating to their actions in response to the alerts. The TAO is designed to record and analyze a wide range of caregiver responses corresponding to the variety of care delivery models and decision protocols that are in use among care providers. Each client and each caregiver in the TAO system becomes the subject of an electronic record which provides quantitative and qualitative information on care delivered and received as well as the impact of these interventions on the care recipient.

Level 2—Care Actions

Since the completion of a TAO is based on an alert generated, the number of TAOs completed depends on the nature of the client and the number of monitoring systems installed at a particular location, i.e., more frail clients will have more alerts, thus generating more TAOs, the more systems installed at a specific location, potentially the more TAOs will be created. Thus, it is not surprising that there is variation in the number of TAOs from one location to another. For example, for a six month period 142 TAOs were recorded at Selfhelp Community Services (New York, USA) with a total of 29 installations, while for a six month period at a Residential Facility for frail elders (London, England) 301 TAOs were produced with a total number of 20 installations and 99 TAOs during a six month period at a Community-based care management organization (London, England) with a total 11 of installations.

The patterns of alerts and care actions, though generally consistent from one Caring Home Site (CHS) to another, do show some interesting variation. The most consistent findings are that for all three locations over 90% of individuals had at least one alert and over 80% had multiple alerts. As for the type of alerts, there were only slight differences among the three locations. For Selfhelp, decline in meal activity is the most frequent alert, followed closely by wake-up and then by general activity, overnight toileting, long bathroom stays, and finally temperature. For the Residential Facility, the frequency pattern was decline in meal activity, overnight toileting, general activity, wake-up, long bathroom stays, and temperature. For the Community-based care management organization, the frequency pattern was decline in meal activity, general activity, wake-up, overnight toileting, long bathroom stays, and temperature.

Differences among the three locations are shown more clearly in the type of actions taken by caregivers. At Selfhelp, where clients live in their own apartments, the most frequent action taken by caregivers was phoning the client to make sure that there was no serious problem. If there was a problem, caregivers' next action was, about equally, either to contact a family member of the client or visit the client. At the Residential Facility, where clients have greater care needs than Selfhelp and live in congregate housing, the initial caregiver action is to visit the client in almost 50% of the cases; while at the Community-based care management organization, where the client needs are the greatest, the most frequent initial action taken is to contact a formal caregiver or family member.

Case Studies

Because of the dynamic nature of outcomes resulting from QuietCare™—they are not discrete events, but unfold over time—it is not possible to reduce them to precisely quantitative results. However, it is possible to illustrate the type of outcomes brought about by the care actions taken by caregivers in response to alerts by three case studies.

The first case study is from Selfhelp and concerns a 95-year-old male living alone. The formal caregiver and the client's daughter simultaneously received alerts indicating a fall in the bathroom. Both responded by immediately going to his apartment, where they found him lying on the bathroom floor. Emergency services were contacted. After EMS personnel examined the client, it was determined that he did not have to be hospitalized, but that he needed to be watched carefully. Since his daughter had not planned to visit her father until the next day, without QuietCare™ his life would have been at risk.

The second case study is from the Community-based care management organization and concerns an 80-year-old female who had a series of activity alerts indicating that the client was leaving her apartment late at night. On one such night, a family member accessed the QuietCare™ website, realized that the client had left, called the Case Manager and searched for the client until finding her, inappropriately dressed, wandering in a neighboring section of London. This incident resulted in support workers staying with the client during the day and relatives sleeping over at night while accelerating the admission process for placement in a residential home. The client has since moved to a residential home which has resulted in "peace of mind for all involved, i.e., the family and the case management team".

The final case study is from the Residential Facility and concerns an 84-year-old male who had three meal alerts within the same week. The caregiver initially spoke to the client by phone, but at the end of the week visited the client to gain a firsthand sense of the situation. The following week, the caregiver brought the case to the attention of other staff at the Residential Facility and contacted the client's physician to develop a plan to both increase the amount of food eaten by the client and to emphasize the importance of eating on a regular schedule. Over the course of the next few days, the caregiver spoke repeatedly with the client about the importance of regular meals and by the following week, the client's eating pattern returned to normal and remained relatively stable over the ensuing months.

Level 3—Informatics

The Third Level involves the use of the data/information produced in Levels 1 and 2, mediated by the TAO, to create information products that track both the individual client who is being monitored and the care delivery system. These information products—named the information management Periodic Automated Care Summary (imPACS)—are produced automatically and can be customized to the specific needs of individuals and organizations. The Wellbeing and Care Tracking Records include charts that track: the number of alerts; the number of TAO response reports; the type and number of actions taken; and the specific outcomes brought about by the actions. In addition, the imPACS system can track staff accountability, provide billable records and through the use of quasi data mining algorithms, produce best practice models, i.e., determine which actions, delivered by what type of caregiver can bring about the most beneficial outcome.

Figure 3 is an example of an Individual Wellbeing Record that summarizes the alerts for and care delivered to a specific client. This record displays the number of alerts and TAOs for the designated time period, provides details about the care delivered and draws attention to any issues that may be of concern—in this example, an increase in overnight toileting. In addition, more details are available at the click of a mouse. Thus, a caregiver, a supervisor, a family member or even the individual being monitored can access more detailed information on each of the categories shown on this first page. This is the prototype of a permanent wellbeing record.

Figure 4 is an example of one component of an Individual Wellbeing Record and depicts the actual meal preparation behavior for an elderly female over a six month period. The number of actual alerts sent by the technology during the same time period is superimposed on the chart. Figure 4 shows a steady decline in meal preparation over the six month period, but there were a surprisingly low number of alerts (7) in these 180 days. This low number of alerts does not reflect the steady decline depicted in the behavioral data and the reason for this appears to be that the day-to-day changes in behavior were too slight to register as significant and thus, to generate an alert, because the alert thresholds were set in such a way that small day-to-day changes in behavior did

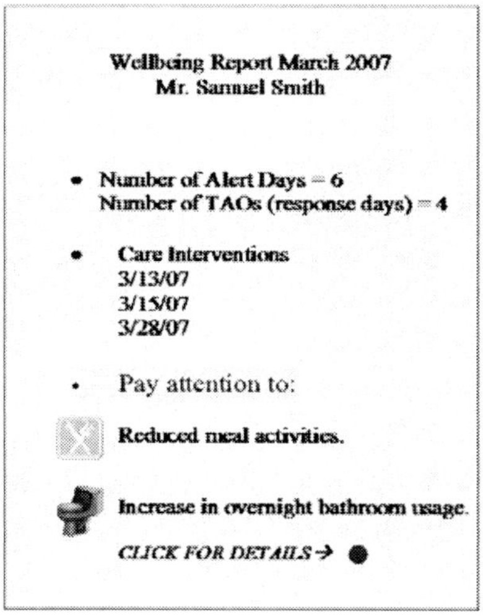
Wellbeing Report March 2007
Mr. Sanmel Smith

- Number of Alert Days = 6
  Number of TAOs (response days) = 4
- Care Interventions
  3/13/07
  3/15/07
  3/28/07
- Pay attention to:

Reduced meal activities.

Increase in overnight bathroom usage.

CLICK FOR DETAILS →

Figure 3: Page 1 of an Individual Wellbeing Report

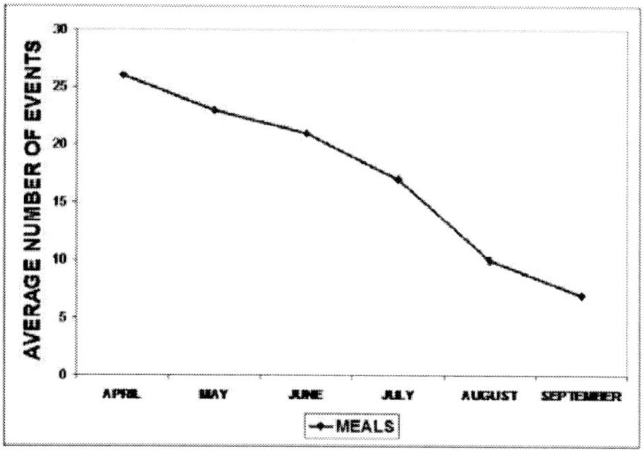

Figure 4: Page 2 of an Individual Wellbeing Report

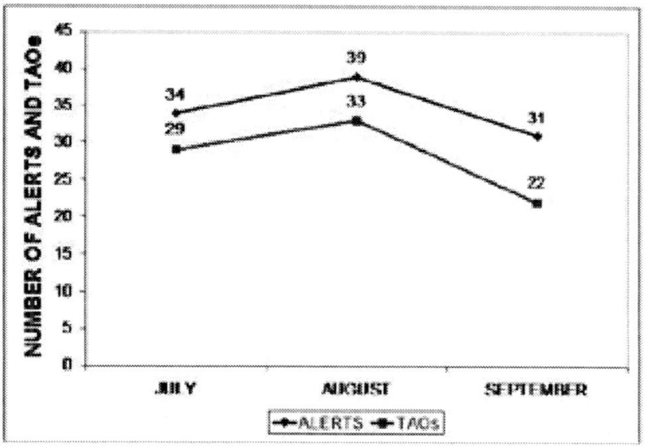

Figure 5: Example of a Care Tracking Record

not generate alerts. This illustrates the challenge in setting alert thresholds. If they are too sensitive, a large number of "false alerts", e.g., indicating a problem when none exists, are generated; if they are too robust, changes in behavior that indicate the onset of some problem may be missed. The thresholds were set to minimize "false positives" so that caregivers are not overwhelmed by alerts that may, over time, be ignored—the cry wolf phenomenon. It is at the informatics level that the subtle changes in behavior that may indicate the emergence of a potential threat to wellbeing are uncovered.

Figure 5 is an example of one component of a Care Tracking Record and depicts the actual events that occurred over a three month period. The lines in the chart show the number of alerts over this period of time versus the number of TAOs that indicated that actions were taken in response to the alerts. Figure 5 appears to show unambiguously that almost 15% of the time the caregiver who received the alerts, did not take a specific action, even though the organization's protocol stated that there had to be a response to each and every alert. On the surface, this discrepancy between the number of alerts and the number of actions recorded on the TAO appears to be a definite violation of this protocol and thus, illustrates how the staff accountability component of the imPACS documents staff negligence. However, in this specific case, there was actually no negligence because the responsible individual had recorded the reasons why no actions were taken in response to the alerts. The TAO form allows the responsible individual to describe the reasons for not taking an action to a specific alert and this information is included in all Care Tracking Records (for illustrative purposes this component of the system was turned off). The following is an actual entry for "no action taken" to an alert indicating a decline in meal preparation on October 24, 2006:

> "Mrs. B. spent yesterday with her daughter and did not eat either lunch or dinner at home. No action was required."

There was a similar entry on the TAOs for each of the alerts for which no action was taken.

From an organizational perspective, the recording of both actions taken and reasons for not taking actions to specific alerts is just good business. Not only does the imPACS document each time an action is taken, thus automatically creating a billable record, but by documenting the reasons for why no action was taken, liability issues are avoided.

Discussion

The findings from the CHI show that not only does behavioral monitoring work, but that the time has come to shift emphasis from the development of increasingly more complex technologies to the development of more effective information products. This does not mean that the technology that is used to collect and transfer the data can be ignored, only that there must be a major shift from the vast expenditures in time and money on the development of ever more sophisticated technology to the development of information products; because Telecare is all about the information: what type, how displayed, how updated, how stored, how retrieved, how used and how paid for. If the information is not usable, then people will not want it and they certainly won't pay for it, regardless of how clever the technology may be.

However, the information products cannot be developed independently of the technology and the care providers. Although the three levels have been discussed separately they are actually part of a single system. Each of the levels can and do operate separately, albeit inefficiently. A technology can operate flawlessly, sending signals to a base station that can transfer the information to a server for analysis, but without someone to receive the information and take action, what is the point. Likewise, a call center can exist, staffed with people who take action and provide care, and there are many such call centers that operate without the type of data/information provided by QuietCare™, e.g., personal emergency response systems. However, in order to take advantage of the more reliable, valid and timely information now available, there must be an integration between these two components. Health informatics exists now, and has for many years, utilizing information from a variety of sources to create, transfer and maintain records on both individuals and groups of varying size. But the advantage derived from integrating the informatics component with the technology and call center components into a single system is compelling.

What specifically are these compelling advantages derived from a fully integrated Telecare system? First, the findings of the CHI show that the information provided by such a system is reliable, valid and most importantly, timely. As each of the three case studies showed, caregivers were alerted to problems—a fall, a decline in eating and risky behavior—which the caregiver could not have known about without QuietCare™. Emergency services were notified, caregivers were able to respond to problems before they became crises and people were able to obtain the level of care they needed. Second, automated, continuously updated, electronic wellbeing records can be generated by the imPACS component of the system. Figure 3 is just the first page of such a wellbeing record. The information provided on this and subsequent pages can be easily customized to the specific care model employed by a care provision company/agency and can be sent electronically to all pertinent caregivers. Finally, the integrated system can also automatically generate continuously updated care delivery records (Figures 4 & 5). Once again, these records can be customized, can be accessed by supervisors and can be used to document services delivered and even play a role in billing.

Conclusion

The main lesson learned from the CHI is that if the goal of Telecare is to produce a product that is intended to be used by caregivers, then integration among the three levels—technology, care and informatics—is essential. However, in practice that means placing less emphasis on technology and much more emphasis on working directly with care providers to incorporate the technology into their existing care model and to produce customized information products. Yes, the technology must work, since if it does not work properly, it cannot be used by caregivers. However, once collaboration begins, there must be continuous on-going assessment of each component and this requires some form of evaluative research. The CHI is one example of this type of evaluative research, but there are others [1] [7]. Who undertakes this research, what role they play in developments at all three levels and where funding is obtained for this research are all important concerns. Once the Telecare is introduced into the real world of care provision, the more difficult it becomes to undertake the evaluative research.

Once again, Barlow, et. al. [4] have clearly articulated both the need for and the challenges associated with such an evidence based evaluative study of Telecare. Since Telecare is a "complex intervention" made up of a number of components that may act both independently and interdependently, "...it is essential to identify all the possible interactions between the different components of the intervention and between the intervention and the setting within which it will be applied in order to develop suitable outcome measures" [4]. In other words, there is an "urgent need for an evaluation 'template' to be developed" for Telecare and it is clear that this template must focus on the interplay between the technology, the actual care delivered and the informatics.

References

[1] Bowes A, & McColgan G. (2006). Smart technology and community care for older people: innovation in West Lothian, Scotland. Age Concern Scotland, Edinburgh, Scotland; 2006.

[2] Brownsell S., Bradley D., Bragg R., Catling P., Carlier J. (2001). An attributable cost model for a telecare system using advanced community alarms. Journal of Telemedicine and Telecare, 7, 63-72.

[3] Cleland J., Louis M., Rigby A., Janssens U, Balk A. (2005). Noninvasive home telemonitoring for patients with heart failure at high risk of recurrent admission and death. Journal of the American College of Cardiology, 45, 1654-1664.

[4] Department of Health. (2006). Updated report of the Evidence Working Group of the Telecare Policy Collaborative chaired by James Barlow – November 2006. Retrieved 12/16/07 from Care Services Improvement Partnership (CSIP) http://www.cat.csip.org.uk/_library/Telecare/CSIP_Factsheet_Telecare_Evidence_13_November_2006.doc

[5] Glascock A. & Kutzik D. (2006). The impact of behavioral monitoring technology on the provision of health care in the home. Journal of Universal Computer Science, 12: 59 – 79.

[6] Kutzik, D., & Glascock, A. (2000). U.S. Patent No. 6,108,685. "System for Generating Periodic Reports, Generating Trend Analysis, and Intervention in Accordance with Trend Analysis from a Detection Subsystem for Monitoring Daily Living Activity—2". Washington, DC. U.S. Patent Office and Trademark Office.

[7] Patel, K. (2006). Development of a new healthcare monitoring system for elderly using emerging communication technologies. Paper presented at IASTED International Conference on Telehealth, Banff, Alberta, Canada

Aging, Disability and Independence
W.C. Mann (Ed.)
IOS Press, 2008

doi:10.3233/978-1-58603-902-8-85

The RoboCare Project: The User's View

Amedeo Cesta[1], Gabriella Cortellessa[1] M. Vittoria Giuliani[2]
Federico Pecora[1], Massimiliano Scopelliti[2] and Lorenza Tiberio[2]
[1]Planning and Scheduling Team
ISTC-CNR, National Research Council of Italy
Institute for Cognitive Science and Technology, Rome (Italy)
[2] Environmental Psychology Unit
ISTC-CNR, National Research Council of Italy
Institute for Cognitive Science and Technology, Rome (Italy)

Abstract: The RoboCare Domestic Environment (RDE) is the result of a three year project aimed at developing cognitive support technology for elderly people. Specifically, the domestic environment is equipped with sensors, intelligent software components and devices which cooperate to provide cognitive support to the assisted person. The RoboCare interaction capabilities have been concentrated in a robotic mediator that acts as the main communication channel between the users and the intelligent domestic environment. This paper presents an evaluation of elder perceptions of assistive robots and smart domestic environments. Results show how the acceptability of robotic devices in home settings does not depend only on the practical benefits they can provide, but also on complex relationships between the cognitive, affective and emotional components of an individual's images of robots. Specifically, we analyzed a number of evaluation criteria related to the robot's appearance, the way in which it communicates with the user, and the perceived usefulness of its support services. Among these criteria, the paper proposes and reports an evaluation of the Proactive interaction modality (where the system takes the initiative) and On-demand interaction (in which the user explicitly requests a service). Users reported the On-demand support services in personal safety scenarios as particularly useful, but less useful in situations which are not critical. The paper also provides a discussion which can be useful for the design of future assistive agents and socially interactive robotic.

Introduction

The use of intelligent technology for supporting elderly people at home has been addressed in various research projects in the last several years [13][14]. These projects have highlighted a number of important issues that need to be addressed: in addition to the problem of coordinating the distributed components, the problem of providing intelligent interaction with the user is undoubtedly among the most critical. A further research area that is gaining attention concerns human-robot interaction for socially assistive applications. There is a need to involve several heterogeneous disciplines in exploring this area [7]. A key aspect of social assistive robots relates to social interactions between human users and robotic agents. For example, Sabanovic et al., [15] emphasized the importance of observation and behavioral analysis of human-robot social interaction in real environments in order to understand the divergent factors in the design of social robots.

This paper describes the RoboCare project whose aim is to create an assistive intelligent environment for older people. The project has involved research groups with different backgrounds with the goal of investigating how intelligent technology for supporting elderly people can improve their quality of life, and maintain their independence at home. The focus on the domestic setting is supported not only by the need for improving the personalization of home technology, but also by recent studies that underscore older people's desire to remain in their homes, and the beneficial effects of increasing their independence at home[8].

As a target domain we have chosen a prototypical home environment where the presence of an intelligent assistant would be of concrete help in the daily life of an elderly person through the integrated performance of advanced distributed components. The most important capability of an intelligent assistant is the continuous maintenance of a high level of situation awareness. This objective is obtained through the interaction of a number of intelligent physical and/or software agents: among others, vision-based sensors, which ensure the acquisition of continuously updated data from the environment; a schedule management software agent, which analyzes the status of every activity being performed within the monitored space; a mobile robotic platform able to behave robustly and continuously in the environment. Specifically, we have incorporated the interaction functionalities on the robotic platform, henceforth called robotic mediator. This entity is an embodied agent whose role is to focus the user's attention in all instances of interaction. Therefore we have concentrated most of the interaction capabilities in the robot, and, additionally, have chosen verbal communication as the main interaction modality. The ultimate goal of the overall system is to provide cognitive support both on-demand, by guaranteeing a real-time question-and-answer service situated to the contextual knowledge of an assisted person, and proactively, by providing an event-driven support grounded on what is going on in a daily

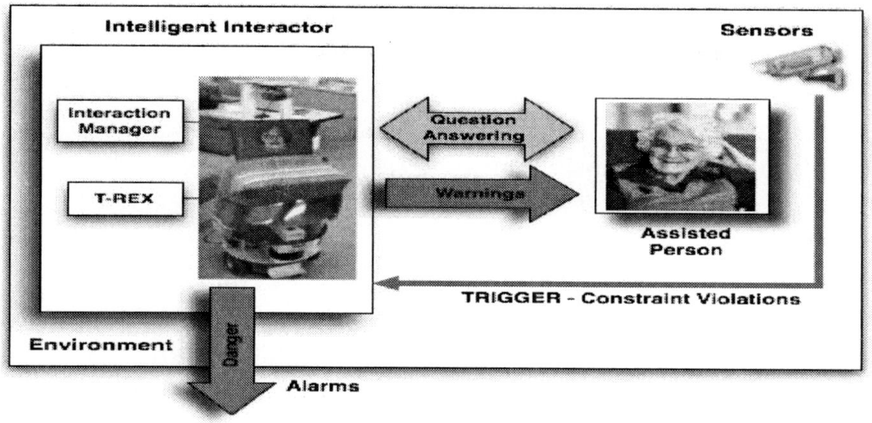

Figure 1: Interactions in the RoboCare environment.

living environment.

How the different interactive functionalities are obtained is described in [6]. In this paper we focus on the evaluation of the tangible robot, analyzing the potential reactions of final users to real life interaction between the elderly person and the robotic agent. We analyze a broad range of features in a controlled experimental setting, focusing on the elder users' evaluation of the system's ability to provide on-demand interactions as well as autonomous system initiative.

We first summarize the key features of the RoboCare domestic environment, emphasizing the role of the robotic mediator and its interaction capabilities. We then describe our user evaluation experiment. We outline the experimental setup, and present the results of the evaluation. The paper ends with a detailed discussion of the results.

The RoboCare Assistive Domain

The RoboCare Domestic Environment (RDE) is the result of a three-year project aimed at developing cognitive support

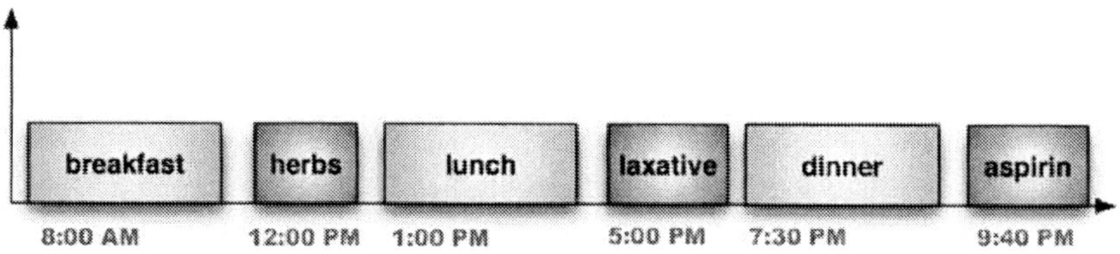

Figure 2: Example of desired behavior specified by the caregiver for the assisted person in form of a schedule

technology for elderly people. Our focus on the domestic scenario stems from a series of studies of different physical environments for older people [4]. The main "actor" in our smart home environment is a robotic agent with verbal interaction capabilities. The interaction content is generated through the combination of different intelligent systems and environmental sensors. A complete description of the technology is given in [5]. Here we present a minimal description that should allow the reader to understand the experimental setup.

The objective of the RDE is to provide support in the management of an older person's daily activities. To this end, the RDE, sketched in Fig. 1, is composed of two fundamental subsystems. One subsystem is an "intelligent observer" of the assisted person: information coming from environmental sensors is used for maintaining an updated representation of what is happening in the environment. The sequence of observations from the artificial vision sensors tracks over time the activities of the observed person. Based on the synthesis of these observations, the system is able to generate a report that reveals when the person's activities have been performed within "reasonable" temporal boundaries or when important anomalies or even violations of their execution have been detected. In this light, the RDE's basic functionality is an example of home Activity Monitor grounded on scheduling technology. On its own, the domestic activity monitor acts as a "silent observer" and does not take initiative with respect to the elder person in any way. On the other hand, the RDE also provides an interface with the assisted elder through an interactive subsystem. This subsystem is essentially a "proactive assistant" which closes the loop between the elder user and the intelligent environment, enabling the system to take initiatives based on Activity Monitor inference.

As a central component for activity management we have employed an AI-based schedule management environment called T-Rex - Tool for schedule representation and execution [12]. T-Rex allows representing a set of activities and their quantitative temporal connections (i.e., a schedule of activities that the user is expected to carry out). These temporal constraints represent the behavioral requirements to which the assisted person should adhere. To be more concrete, let us consider a behavioral pattern described by a schedule composed of 6 different activities (breakfast, lunch, dinner, as well as taking three different medicines). Due to medical requirements, let us also suppose that such activities must satisfy certain temporal requirements, such as "dinner should not begin before 7:30 PM, nor should it occur less than 5 hours after lunch" and "aspirin should only be taken after dinner, but not too late", and so on.

An "ideal schedule", i.e., an enactment of these activities that does not violate any temporal constraint, is shown in Fig. 2. Broadly speaking, the objective of the Activity Monitor is to recognize deviations from this ideal situation. Specifically, the system should assess the extent to which the user's behavior deviates from this situation. This equates to assessing which temporal constraints are progressively violated during the day. In summary, system interventions are driven by constraint violations: warnings, alarms and suggestions result from violated constraints. System interventions are processed by the interactive subsystem on board the robotic mediator.

Managing Interaction with the User

As already mentioned, interaction within RoboCare relies on an embodied robotic assistant as the focal point between the user and the system. Communication between the user and the robotic mediator occurs verbally. For the purposes of this study, we distinguish two forms of interaction based on who takes the initiative to start a dialogue:

(1) On-Demand interaction in which the user takes the initiative first. The assisted person commences interaction, for instance, by querying the system's knowledge base: "have I taken my pills?" or "can I make an appointment for tomorrow at 5 PM?"

(2) Proactive interaction in which the intelligent environment commences interaction guided by its internal reasoning. Within RoboCare, constraint violations have been considered as a trigger for the system to take the initiative and perform some actions: issue an alarm in case of illness, or verbalize warnings and suggestions.

Our work explicitly focuses on the development of active and, at the same time, unobtrusive services to integrate within the artificial assistant. All interaction services rely on the Interaction

Manager. This module essentially consists of a rule-based system that fires situation-action rules. In other words, it continuously assesses the situation and activates a particular sub-module as an action.

The main "interaction occasions" managed in the current version of the intelligent assistant are also shown in Fig. 1. We categorize as On-Demand interaction the "Question/Answer" category of dialogues. This activity is triggered by a speech input from the assisted person. The generation of the answer is managed mostly internally to the manager who has information on activity history and/or on the current state of the environment, to answer questions like "Have I had lunch?" or "What time is it?"

Instances of Proactive interaction are "Danger" and "Warning" scenarios. Undoubtedly, one of the important tasks for assistance is to recognize emergencies for the monitored person. The emergency trigger is fired by particular combinations of the input provided by the sensors that monitor the environment and the assisted person. As an example we can discriminate as a dangerous situation the case in which a person is "lying down on the kitchen floor" or "lying down in bed half and hour after usual wake up", rather than "lying down in bed within an expected period" which is recognized as a regular situation. The danger trigger is dealt with by a specific behavior of the multi-agent system that interrupts the usual flow of activities and undertakes an action: the robot is sent to the assisted person, a specific dialogue is attempted, and if no answer from the assisted person is obtained, an Alarm is immediately fired to the external world (such as a call to a relative, to an emergency help desk).

A warning scenario is one in which constraint violations are detected by the T-Rex activity monitor. Broadly speaking, the activity monitor decides the values for the variables that are used by the interaction manager to trigger a proactive dialogue with the assisted person. The content of the dialogue is synthesized on the basis of the monitor's internal knowledge.

Overall the Interaction Manager in Fig. 1 is a quite simple planner that supervises the initiative of the "interactor" towards the assisted person. It is worth underscoring how the combination of this manager and the activity monitor endows the whole assistive environment with capabilities of proactive participation in a mixed-initiative interaction.

Experiments with Elder Users

The remainder of this paper describes our experiments aimed at understanding the perception of older people towards the assistance that the robot (and thus the assistive environment as a whole) is able to offer at the moment.

Previous Evaluations

A previous study [17], performed at the beginning of the RoboCare project, was aimed at drawing some preliminary wishes and requirements for assistive robots. This evaluation analyzed laypeople's representations of domestic robots with respect to a variety of topics: the users' expectations of the robot's capabilities to perform different everyday activities at home; their emotional response to a domestic robot; the image of the robot, referring to shape, size, color, cover material, speed; preferences and expectancies about the robot's personification (given name, etc.) and the modalities of human-robot communication and interaction.

People overestimate manipulative abilities and underestimate cognitive capabilities of the robot, whose representation is somewhat unrealistic: domestic robots are still too far away from everyday life experience of lay people. In addition, people of different ages showed very divergent opinions and preferences. In particular, older people clearly indicated a preference for a small robot, hardly resembling a human being, minimally intrusive in personal and domestic life; not autonomously free to move in the domestic environment, and simply responsive to tasks that needed to be performed. While its practical utility was recognized, the robot emerged as a potential source of danger and discomfort in private life, and the idea of a non-autonomous device seemed to be a way to ward off anxiety. Another issue to be addressed has to do with the context in which the robot is expected to operate. The use of new technologies and domestic robots in the home environment is not only a matter of general human-technology interaction, but is also associated with the specific sphere of human life in which assistance is needed [16]. Elderly people showed a rather positive attitude towards a technological modification in the domestic environment, yet the inclination to use technological devices is strongly associated with their individual difficulties in doing activities. In some situations, a technological aid seemed to be unrealistic, or unpractical, or it would have better been replaced by a more common alternative. In other cases, concerning health and personal/environmental safety above all, it emerged as a suitable solution to address limitations that resulted from impairments.

The Present Study

The previously mentioned studies focused on users' attitudes toward a purely imaginary robotic agent, with unspecified abilities and not operating in a real domestic environment. For this reason, differences in users' reactions could have been related to both diverse knowledge and bias toward technologies.

The final prototype achieved by RoboCare overcame this limitation. The evaluation of a tangible robot eliminates preconceptions and other biases. Performing the evaluation on the RDE prototype allows us to draw specific conclusions on the prototype itself, and also to investigate some general issues relative to the challenges of assistive technology for elderly people. This analysis is in line with current recommendations for the evaluation of complex assistive technology. For instance, Hutchins [9] recognized that human-robot interaction should be evaluated on socio-culturally constituted activities outside the design laboratory. In this light, the aim of our research is to analyze the potential reactions of older persons to real life interactions with an assistive robot.

The present analysis considered eight different scenarios, which were meant to be representative of daily situations in which older people may be involved. The situations were selected with reference to previous research on this topic [17], ranging from the most emotionally involving to less critical and emotionally neutral, with the aim of exploring elderly people's evaluations of the potential role of a domestic robot as a useful support. Specifically, the study focused on three main aspects.

First, we performed an evaluation of how meaningful each scenario is with respect to the respondents' every day life. This allows us to understand how useful state-of-the-art assistive technology can be in real situations. Moreover, it provides an indication as to whether we are employing this technology to solve real needs. Scenarios were arranged so the robot would be evaluated in different types of interactive situations: we propose a main distinction between "On-demand" and "Proactive" scenarios. On-demand scenarios imply an explicit request for the robot's activity by the final user; in proactive scenarios, the robot autonomously intervenes in the domestic environment, for both an emergency and to provide suggestions. By comparing the On-demand and Proactive situations, we sought to determine the elder's preferred level of autonomy for the robot.

Second, we focused on the respondents' assessment of our robotic mediator, including the physical appearance of the robot, its interaction capabilities, and its suitability in the domestic context (size, mobility, integration with the environment).

Third, we observed user preferences with respect to robot's features in simulating a human. Although our robot is not anthropomorphic, it is possible to deploy it in two slightly different versions: one in which the robot has a 3D facial representation (whose lip movement is synchronized with the speech synthesizer), and one without a facial representation. These variants were used to toggle the variable "Similarity to human beings", which emerged as a key component in elderly people's representation of domestic robots [17].

Materials

Eight short movies (ranging from about 30 seconds to little more than one minute) were developed showing potential interaction scenarios between an elderly person and the RDE's robotic agent in a real domestic environment (see Fig. 4) .

The features of the robotic agent were manipulated according to two different experimental conditions: in the first condition ("Face") a robot showing a human speaking face on a notebook monitor; in the second ("No-face"), a robot with no reference to human features (see Figure 3). The eight scenarios presented everyday life situations in which the robot provides cognitive support to the elderly person, and referred to critical areas, as highlighted by previous research: (a) management of personal/environmental safety, (b) healthcare, (c) reminding events/deadlines, (d) support to activity planning, (e) suggestions. In the following, the eight scenarios are shortly described.

Scenario 1 [Environmental safety]

The actor/actress is sitting on the sofa, watching TV. In the meantime, in the kitchen the sauce on the stove is overcooking. The sensors communicate this information to the robot. As a consequence, the robot moves toward the actor/actress and says: "The pot is burning. You should turn it off". The actor/actress immediately goes to the kitchen and turns off the stove.

Scenario 2 [Personal safety]

The actor/actress is sitting on the sofa, reading a magazine. Suddenly, he/she feels ill, and faints. The camera recognizes the situation and communicates this information to the robot. The robot approaches the actor/actress and says: "Are you all right?". As it gets no answer, the robot calls the actor's/actress' son at work, who calls the medical emergency. The final scene shows the son and the doctor in the living room with the actor/actress, who feels fine.

Scenario 3 [Finding objects]

The actor/actress is sitting on the sofa, and takes a magazine to read. Suddenly, he/she realizes that the glasses are not on the table in front of him/her. The actor/actress calls the robot and asks: "Where are my glasses?". The sensors in the rooms search for the glasses, and finally find them in the kitchen. The robot answers: "The glasses are on the table in the kitchen". The actor/actress goes to the kitchen and takes the glasses, then goes back to the sofa and starts reading the magazine.

Scenario 4 [Reminding analyses]

The actor/actress is in the kitchen. He/she is about to have breakfast. When he/she puts the pot on the stove to warm up the milk, the robot says: "You cannot have breakfast now. You have

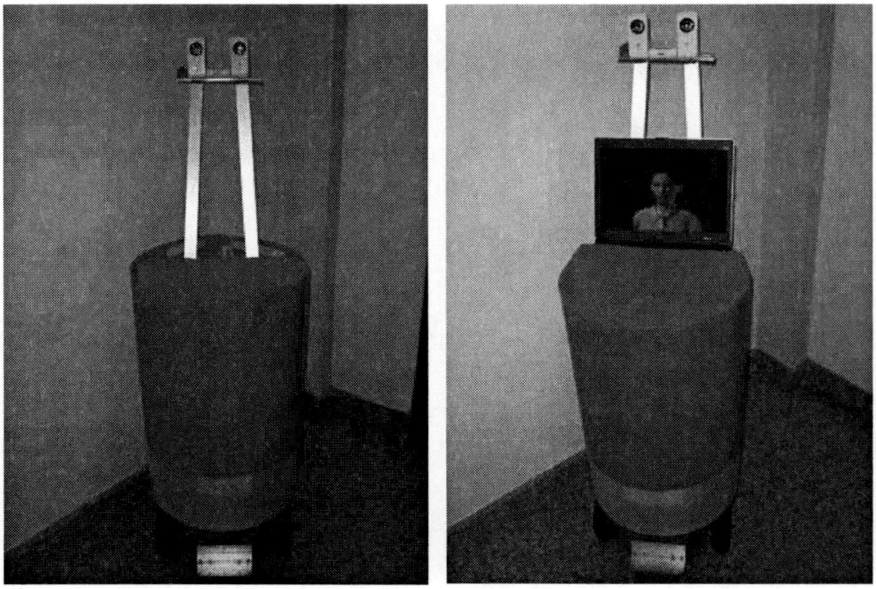

Figure 3: The two experimental conditions of the robot.

an appointment for a medical analysis". The actor/actress answers: "You're right. I had forgotten all about it!"

Scenario 5 [Activity planning]

The actor/actress is on the phone in the living room. He/she is speaking to the secretary of a clinical center to get an appointment for a medical examination. The secretary proposes an appointment for the next day, with two alternatives: either in the morning, or in the afternoon. The actor/actress asks the robot for eventual engagements the following day. The robot answers: "You have another engagement in the morning. In the afternoon, you do not have any appointments". The actor/actress accepts the appointment in the afternoon.

Scenario 6 [Reminding medication]

The actor/actress is sleeping on the sofa, and suddenly wakes up. He/she does not realize what time is it, and thus he/she asks the robot. The robot answers: "It is four o'clock". The actor/actress does not remember whether or not he/she took his/her medicine after lunch, and asks the robot. The robot answers: "Yes, you took you medicine."

Scenario 7 [Suggestions]

The actor/actress is watching TV on the sofa. It is five o'clock. The robot enters the living room and says: "You have been

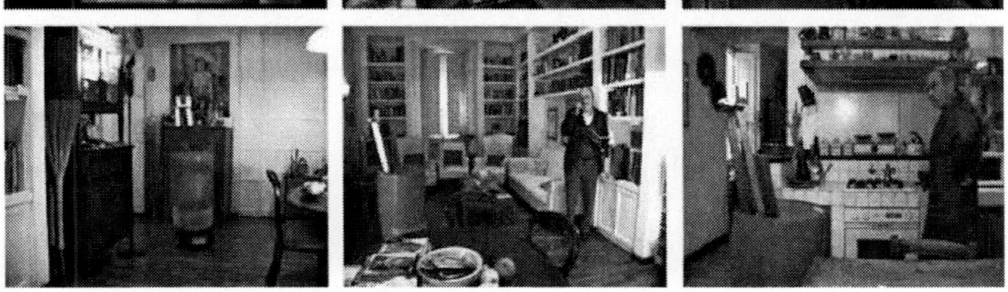

Figure 4: Sample frames from the videos depicting the eight scenarios

spending all the day at home. Why don't you go out and have a walk?". The actor/actress answers: "I really don't feel like it... I think I'll go water the plants in the garden".

Scenario 8 [Reminding events]

The actor/actress is having breakfast in the kitchen. The robot reminds him/her: "Today it's your friend Giovanni's birthday. Remember to call him". The actor/actress answers: "You are right. I will do it right away". Then he/she goes to the living room and calls Giovanni.

Scenarios 1, 2 and 4 illustrate proactive situations referring to domestic healthcare and emergencies; scenarios 7 and 8 feature proactive situations implying suggestions; scenarios 3, 5 and 6 illustrate on-demand interactions.

Tools

A questionnaire was developed for data collection. It consisted of three sections, plus a final part for socio-demographics. The sections were arranged as follows:

> *Section 1.* Eight fill-in papers, each of them referring to one of the eight scenarios, were presented. For each scenario, questions were asked about the likelihood of the situation for the elderly person, and the utility and acceptability of the robot.
>
> *Section 2.* An attitude scale, consisting of 45 Likert-type items, referring to the physical aspect of the robot, its behavior and communication modalities; the level of integration with the domestic environment; the degree of perceived intrusion/disturbance of the robot in everyday life and routines; the personal advantages and disadvantages of having such a device at home.
>
> *Section 3.* An emotional scale, consisting of sixteen adjectives through which respondents have to evaluate the possible presence of the robot in their home.

In the Likert-type items, the respondents had to express their level of agreement/disagreement on a scale ranging from 0 ("I totally disagree") to 4 ("I completely agree").

Participants and procedure

Participants included forty people, 13 male and 27 female, ranging in age from 56 to 88 years, with a mean age of 70.3 years. Participants educational level was as follows: 17.9% attended primary school, 43.6% attended middle school, 25.6% attended high school, 12.9% have a degree. Most (82.5%) were retired. Before retirement, 22.5% were teachers, 15% were office workers. Subjects were randomly assigned to one of the two experimental conditions (Face/No-face). The movies were either projected on a notebook monitor, in a face-to-face administration, or on a larger screen, in a small-group administration. Two different sequences of scenario presentation were used to avoid the potential influence of an order effect of episodes on results. After viewing each scenario, participants were asked to complete Section 1 of the questionnaire. At the end of the whole presentation, subjects were asked to give general evaluations of the robot (Sections 2-3 of the questionnaire), and to fill the final section of the questionnaire which addressed socio-demographics.

Results

The results were obtained from a combination of quantitative (ANOVA, c2 and Pearson's correlation) and qualitative analyses of the user evaluation questionnaires.

On-demand vs. Proactive scenarios

An analysis of meaningfulness of scenarios shows that our selection was effective in identifying typical everyday situations. On the whole, both On-demand and Proactive situations involving emergency and healthcare were evaluated as significantly more common than Proactive situations referring to suggestions [2] in Proactive situations involving emergency and healthcare the robot was evaluated as significantly more useful than in On-demand and Proactive situations referring to suggestions; [3] finally, the preference

Table 1: Evaluation of the different types of situations. Users were asked to evaluate on a scale from 0 to 4.

Type of situation	Meaningfulness		Usefulness		Preference	
	Mean	*St. dev.*	*Mean*	*St. dev.*	*Mean*	*St. dev.*
Proactive (Emergency)	2.51^a	.59	2.74^a	.73	2.48^a	.87
On-demand	2.53^a	.67	2.44^b	.85	2.13^b	.97
Proactive (Suggestions)	1.99^b	.83	1.94^c	.98	1.76^c	1.13

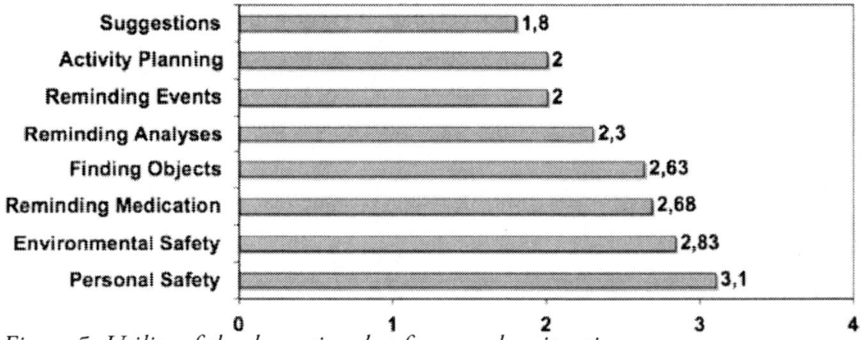

Figure 5: Utility of the domestic robot for everyday situations.

for the robot's support was significantly higher in Proactive situations involving emergency and healthcare than in On-demand and Proactive situations referring to suggestions [4] (see Tab. 1).

A global picture of the robotic mediator reveals a rather positive perception. The robot emerged as a very useful device for Personal and Environmental safety, Reminding medications, and Finding objects but not particularly useful in the case of Suggestions (see Fig. 5).

In addition to utility, the robot was also indicated as a solution that users would accept when difficulties arise, again with specific reference to Personal ($M = 2.95$, $sd = 1.06$) and Environmental safety ($M = 2.55$, $sd = 1.01$). In general, a significant correlation emerged (Pearson's r) between meaningfulness of a specific scenario, utility of and preference for the robot in that scenario (i.e., the higher the meaningfulness of the scenario, the higher the users' perceived utility and the probability they would accept such a device at home).

General evaluation of the robot.

As to the different characteristics of the robot, some Positive and Negative aspects emerged (see Tab. 2).

Positive Aspects

Both face-to-face interaction with people and communication modality were on average positively assessed; in addition, elderly people favorably evaluated interactions with the robot for training to reduce loss of cognitive functioning. The overall integration with the home environment was viewed positively, even though total freedom of movement was not completely appreciated. Advantages of having a robot in the domestic environment include feeling safer, providing support for cognitive functioning and, in general, organizing everyday activities.

Table 2: General evaluation of the robot

Positive Aspects	Mean	St. dev.
Face-to-face interaction	2,60	1,23
Communication modality	2,33	,62
Cognitive Training	2,53	1,24
Integration	2,34	,91
People feel safer	3,23	1,14
Support for activities	2,98	1,03
Negative Aspects	*Mean*	*St. dev.*
Managment difficulty	2,95	1,11
Economic costs	3,25	,84
Possible Dependance	2,48	1,45

Negative Aspects

Difficulties with the management of the device (such as need for repairs) and the possible economic costs are expected. Also, users seemed to worry about the potential to become dependent on the robot in certain cognitive tasks. The emotional reaction of elderly people to the robot was very good, scoring high on the positive adjectives useful, interesting and relaxing, and scoring very low on the negative adjectives scary, overwhelming, gloomy, dangerous, uncontrollable (see Fig. 6).

Similarity to human beings

The No-face version of the robot was preferred significantly more, appearing both less mechanical and less cold. The No-face version was also evaluated as having a significantly higher level of integration with the domestic environment and a larger variety of advantages than the Face version, referring to ease of use and a low need for repair[5]. In addition, elderly people seemed to be more likely to develop a psychological attachment towards the No-face version than towards the Face version [6].

Discussion

This study addressed some general acceptability requirements for assistive robotic agents. The general framework depicted by

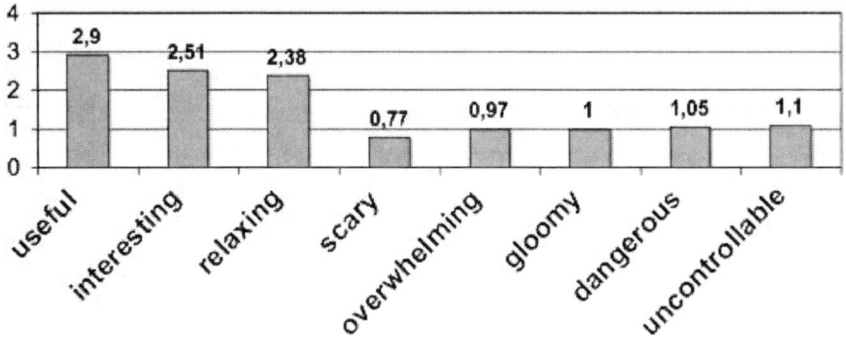

Figure 6: Emotional reaction of elder people to the robot (Means)

the On-demand vs. Proactive situations emerged to be highly meaningful in elderly people's experience, and the evaluation of proposed scenarios plainly shows their main concerns in everyday life and the potential role of a domestic robot in supporting them. Elderly people perceive a clear distinction between important and unimportant activities to be performed at home. For those activities which are perceived of greatest relevance, mainly concerning personal and environmental safety, the autonomy of the robot in the management of the home environment and in taking decisions proved to be a very useful resource. The robot is also appreciated for its capability in responding to a specific need expressed by the user, especially when referring to a cognitive difficulty associated with ageing, and involving activities related to healthcare (e.g., remembering things to do or what has been already done, with particular reference to medications and analyses).

Conversely, a robot making suggestions regarding unimportant activities is perceived as somewhat irritating. A well-defined relationship between likelihood of situations, perceived utility of and preference for the robot emerged. In the situation involving an emergency the preference for the robotic support was higher than the perceived likelihood of the situation itself, and the perception of utility scores highest. Conversely, with respect to activities that are not considered to be essential in everyday life, older people had a tendency to assign a low score on likelihood of occurrence, and even lower scores on usefulness and preference.

Overall, even if emergencies are not likely to occur, their central role in elderly people's experience makes the perceived utility of and the expressed preference towards a proactive robot higher. This picture is in line with the model of successful aging put forward by, which stresses the role of selection and optimization of activities with increasing age, and the importance of compensation strategies to manage the loss of personal resources.

Our findings differ with Scopelliti [16] in that we found older people are not afraid of the robot's autonomy, when they can actually understand what a robot can do in the domestic environment. In other words, a representation grounded on unrealistic ideas (as the ones proposed by science fiction) may negatively bias attitudes and expectations.

The overall evaluation of the robot emerged to be very positive, with reference to many specific features, ranging from interaction modalities to the degree of integration in the domestic environment. In this respect, however, the issue of safety confirmed to play a key role in elderly people's experience and, though not anxious about it, they would like the robot to move in the domestic environment only when a specific task has to be performed.

The most distinctive feature of the robot was undoubtedly associated with its practical utility, as emerged from both a cognitive and an affective evaluation. The robot can help people in the management of everyday activities requiring an efficient cognitive functioning. In addition, the presence of such a device in the domestic environment appears to be fundamental in making elderly people feel safer, especially when they live alone. On the other hand, older people were aware of potential difficulties with the robot, for both practical and psychological reasons. The practical difficulties are related to expenses, both to acquire the assistive robot and to maintain it. More importantly from a psychological point of view, older people seem to forecast a potential loss in personal autonomy and a dependence on the robot, which might reduce their competence and self-efficacy [3], key factors for successful ageing [10][11] [18]. In this respect, they appreciated the opportunity to interact with the robot not only passively, but also through active training to enhance their cognitive functioning. Their attitude (affective aspect) about the robot was definitely positive, being in terms of relaxation and interest; in addition, the robot was not considered a source of danger, fear or other negative affects.

The physical aspect of the robot emerged as an important feature that impacts acceptability. Any representation of the robot as a human being seemed to have a negative impact on their feeling about the robot. The No-face version of the robot was definitely preferred, and the physical aspect proved to also affect the evaluation of other unrelated features. The No-face version was perceived as less artificial and psychologically distant from the user, better integrated in the home setting and easier to manage. In other words, the better the aspect, the stronger the perception of positive qualities attributed to the robot. This suggests a halo effect, consistently emerging in social sciences with reference to personality judgments (e.g., [1]).

Open Issues

Given its exploratory purposes, there were limitations with this study. First, our preliminary results emerged from a small sample, and a stronger statistical robustness is needed. Our study presumably lacks external validity in that our respondents were generally well-educated and healthy: the evaluation of a robotic agent which has to be a support for impairments related to ageing may be different when people are more in need. Nonetheless, our findings can be considered as a starting point relative to acceptability of robotic agents in the homes of older persons. Older persons perceived the robot as a practical device: they do not seem to be particularly interested in matters of aspect, shape, cover materials; and they prefer that it not resembles a human being. On the other hand, interaction which involves a face-to-face relationship seemed to reduce a feeling of emotional distance from this device. It would be interesting to evaluate in future research a possible difference in response to a domestic assistive device which cannot move about in the environment. An environmental system equipped with software, sensory and speaking services would probably be able to perform the same activities provided by the mobile device shown in this study. At the time of writing, we have initiated experimentation with a system that does not employ a robotic mediator for interaction. It communicates with the domestic environment through pervasive microphones and speakers. The aim of this further study is to understand how acceptability might be affected by such a difference.

Acknowledgements
This research is partially supported by MIUR (Italian Ministry of Education, University and Research) under project ROBOCARE (A Multi-Agent System with Intelligent Fixed and Mobile Robotic Components). Special thanks to the colleagues of the Dept. of Computer and Systems Science (DIS) of the University of Rome "La Sapienza" for joint work on the RoboCare intelligent environment.

Footnotes

[1]At the moment sensors are cameras whose observation are elaborated by artificial vision algorithms to extract useful features.

[2]$(F(2,78) = 15.00, p < .001)$

[3]$(F(2,78) = 27.84, p < .001)$

[4]$(F(2,78) = 20.83, p < .001)$

[5]overall preference: $(F(1,38) = 6.34, p < .05)$; less mechanical $(F(1,38) = 5.11, p < .05)$; less cold: $(F(1,38) = 7.25, p < .05)$; better integrated: $(F(1,38) = 5.65, p < .05)$; ease of use: $(F(1,38) = 9.36, p < .01)$; low need for repair: $(F(1,38) = 4.33, p < .05)$

References

[1] Asch, S. (1946) Forming impressions of personality. Journal of Abnormal and Social Psychology (41):258-290.

[2] Baltes, P. B., and Baltes, M. M. (1990) Psychological Perspectives on Successful Aging: The Model of Selecive Optimization with Compensation. New York: Cambridge Univ. Press. 1-34.

[3] Bandura, A. (1977) Self-efficacy: Toward a unifying theory of behavioural change. Psychological Review 84:191-215.

[4] Cesta, A., and Pecora, F. (2006) Integrating Intelligent Systems for Elder Care in RoboCare. In Mann, W., and Helal, A., eds., Promoting Independence for Older Persons with Disabilities. IOS Press. 65-73.

[5] Cesta, A.; Cortellessa, G.; Pecora, F.; and Rasconi, R. (2007a) Coordinating Heterogeneous Agents to Synthesize Proactive Monitoring. In ICAPS Workshop on Planning and Plan Execution for Real-World Systems, Providence, RI, USA.

[6] Cesta, A.; Cortellessa, G.; Pecora, F.; and Rasconi, R. (2007b) Supporting Interaction in the RoboCare Intelligent Assistive Environment. In Proccedings of AAAI Spring Symposium on Interaction Challenges for Intelligent Assistants.

[7] Feil-Seifer, D., and Mataric', M. J. (2005) Defining socially assistive robotics. In Proc. 9th Int. Conf. on Rehabilitation Robotics (ICORR-05), 465-468. IEEE.

[8] Giuliani, M.; Scopelliti, M.; and Fornara, F. (2005) Elderly people at home: technological help in everyday activities. In IEEE International Workshop on Robot and Human Interactive Communication (ROMAN 2005), 365-370.

[9] Hutchins, E. (1995) Cognition in the Wild. MIT Press.

[10] Lawton, M. P. (1982) Time budgets of older people: A window on four lifestyles. Journal of Gerontology 37:115-123.

[11] McAvay, G. J.; Seeman, T. E.; and Rodin, J. (1996) A longitudinal study of change in domain-specific self-efficacy among older adults. Journal of Gerontology 51:243-253.

[12] Pecora, F.; Rasconi, R.; Cortellessa, G.; and Cesta, A. (2006) User-Oriented Problem Abstractions in Scheduling, Customization and Reuse in Scheduling Software Architectures. Innovations in Systems and Software Engineering 2(1):1-16

[13] Pineau, J.; Montemerlo, M.; Pollack, M.; Roy, N.; and Thrun, S. (2003) Towards Robotic Assistants in Nursing Homes: Challenges and Results. Robotics and Autonomous Systems 42(3-4):271-281.

[14] Pollack, M. (2005) Intelligent Technology for an Aging Population:The Use of AI to Assist Elders with Cognitive Impairment. AI Magazine 26(2):9-24.

[15] Sabanovic, S., Michalowski, M. P., Simmons, R. (2006) Robots in the wild: Observing human-robot social interaction outside the lab. In 9th IEEE International Workshop on Advanced Motion Control (pp. 596 - 601). Istanbul: IEEE

[16] Scopelliti, M.; Giuliani, M. V.; D'Amico, A. M.; and Fornara, F. (2004) If I had a robot ... peoples' representation of domestic robots. In Keates, S.; Clarkson, P. J.; Langdon, P. M.; and Robinson, P., eds., Design for a more inclusive world. London: Springer-Verlag. 257-266.

[17] Scopelliti, M.; Giuliani, M. V.; and Fornara, F. (2005) Robots in a domestic setting: A psychological approach. Universal Access in the Information Society 4(2):146-155.

[18] Willis, S. L. (1996) Everyday cognitive competence in elderly persons: Conceptual issues and empirical findings. The Gerontologist 36:595-601.

Aging, Disability and Independence
W.C. Mann (Ed.)
IOS Press, 2008

doi:10.3233/978-1-58603-902-8-105

Living Labs: Helping to Meet the Needs of Ageing People?

Brendan Galbraith[1], Maurice Mulvenna[2], Suzanne Martin[3], Eileen McGloin[4]
[1]Business Organisation and Management, University of Ulster, Northern Ireland; [2]School of Computing and Mathematics, University of Ulster, Northern Ireland; [3]School of Health Sciences, University of Ulster, Northern Ireland; [4]ECMG Consulting Limited, Belfast, Northern Ireland

Abstract: This paper introduces a new enabling method for open innovation, called living labs. Living labs are spaces where companies, public organizations such as councils or health and welfare organizations and communities can work together to develop and prototype new products, technologies and services in real environments embedded in the community or market place. We describe the steps being taken to establish a living lab in Northern Ireland, called TRAIL (Technologies for Rurality, Ageing and Independent Living). The objective of TRAIL, achieved through community-facilitated and user-driven studies, is to create service and product innovations that will enable rural and ageing citizens to live independently in the heart of their communities. TRAIL will develop pilot products and services for this sector of the community, with the added benefit of validating and fine-tuning the innovation methods. Importantly, TRAIL will support a fusion of innovation models, technology and integrated community care-based approaches.

Introduction

Global population growth is being impacted by the rising percentage of older persons, and this is a trend that will continue for the foreseeable future. We now face the challenge of healthcare service initiatives being driven by the goals of individual autonomy and quality of life. Around 30% of the European population will be over 60 by 2020. Approximately 100,000 more older people will be living alone in Ireland than in 2004. This demographic change will pose increased problems for health and social care systems. The challenge is to change the type of care provision for increasing numbers of older people, such as freeing hospital beds more quickly, to decrease overall costs.

Delivering services to individuals in their own home enables people to maintain their independence. It is where successful service delivery is more likely to be most cost-effective but it also brings new challenges. Helping those with chronic diseases, for example, COPD, Diabetes, and Alzheimer's disease, to live independently at home will require the increased and sustained application of information and communication technology.

In this paper, we present an emerging European user-focused and open innovation model, Living Labs, and then proceed to outline the fledgling Living Lab in Northern Ireland - TRAIL (Technologies for Rurality, Ageing and Independent Living).

The Rationale for a Living Lab

In Europe, the Finnish EU Presidency has recently launched a new Public-Private-Partnership (PPP) innovation model called the European Network of Living Labs (ENOLL). ENOLL aims to be a fundamental step towards connecting the Lisbon Strategy (EU goal of becoming the most dynamic and competitive knowledge-based economy in the world by 2010) to a new and more user-driven European Innovation System. It applies new methodologies for co-creative research and innovation, including new means of Intellectual Property (IP) development, management of research and innovation as well as new forms for direct user involvement in the innovation process. Further, the chair of the ENOLL and director of research, Nokia, Veli-Pekka Niitamo [5] describes Living Labs as:

> *"an emerging Public Private Partnership (PPP) where firms, public authorities and people work together with creating, prototyping, validating and testing new services, businesses, markets and technologies in real-life contexts, such as cities, city regions, rural areas and collaborative virtual networks between public and private players."*

Essentially, Living Labs are community-facilitated, open and user-driven interventions.

The Rationale for a Living Lab in Ireland

The University of Ulster will make a significant contribution to the living lab concept through its TRAIL initiative. TRAIL represents a developing Public-Private Partnership (PPP) where companies, public authorities and communities work together creating, prototyping, validating and testing new services, businesses, markets and technologies in real-life contexts in the regions, rural areas and virtual spaces between public and private players in the region of the North of Ireland. It is our strategic intention to collaborate further with our existing international networks and to integrate fully our activities with ENOLL members and other international clusters.

In practical terms, the introduction of the Living Labs will be challenging, given the post-conflict climate of weak North of Ireland high-tech performance and co-operation. There is an extreme need to introduce fresh thinking. A new PPP Northern Ireland innovation model can perhaps, be better understood by examining three further weaknesses of the general EU innovation system; (1) the causes of the underperforming venture capital (VC) industry (especially early-stage funding) (2) the relatively small high-tech industrial sector and low levels of innovative enterprises and (3) the low levels of cooperation between innovative enterprises and customers, universities and public research institutes. Moreover, the Nobel economics laureate, Robert Mundell, posits that another key EU challenge for innovators is that the expanding ageing population does not pick up the new technology and growth innovations as rapidly as others. We feel that this challenge is mirrored by great opportunity. Namely, the demographic changes will inevitably pose increased problems for social security and healthcare systems and in turn, create significant opportunities for researchers, entrepreneurs and other stakeholders. TRAIL and the University of Ulster in its capacity as the largest university on the island of Ireland is fully committed to playing a full role in the community-driven (business, citizens, public sector agencies and academia) economic and social development of Northern Ireland.

The University of Ulster has a vision to be a model of an outstanding regional university with a national and international reputation for quality. Sharing best practice, gained through world-class research activity and excellence in teaching, with business and the community is an essential part of this mission. Further, the University of Ulster (UU) has over the past decade helped facilitate the technological commercialization and the expansion of Northern Ireland's evolving innovation ecosystem by its extensive support and investment of UU science parks, incubators and research institutes. The TRAIL innovation model aims to further capitalize on this infrastructure and improve levels of co-operation (especially university and industry links) and the quality of technology transfer mechanisms. This is very timely as it links with a core strategic aim of the University of Ulster to "establish the University as a sector leader in promoting creativity and innovation". Key to this are open innovation models like TRAIL which has established co-operation among users and key stakeholders including business, community, multidisciplinary academia and research institutions, and government agencies and rural areas which are key drivers of the TRAIL Living Labs model.

The TRAIL vision is to develop participative methods that identify the unmet health-related needs of ageing, rural dwellers of Northern Ireland and the border counties of Ireland as they age in place. The objectives are to identify and prioritize unmet user needs, identify opportunities to address these unmet needs using knowledge and technology transfer activities and subsequently develop pilot products, solutions and services that address the unmet need, in partnership with Health and Welfare Organizations (HWO), indigenous enterprises, and ageing, rural people themselves.

Embracing the open and mutually collaborative nature of the Living Labs model, TRAIL expects to gain and contribute international knowledge and method exchange opportunities with extant living labs as well as the sharing of participatory and appreciative action research, validations and development of participative and user-centered methods as applied to ageing and rural people in Ireland to the broader European base of older citizens. This international collaborative ethos is in line with the renewed innovation thinking by major international companies. Chesborough [1] compares companies such as DuPoint, Merck, IBM, GE and AT&T, who, not long ago, were viewed as being leaders due to their significant internal research and development programmes, to the strong competition they are facing today by newer companies. The newer companies, Intel, Microsoft, Sun, Oracle, Cisco, Genetech, Amgen, Genzyme, have been very innovative, but they achieved their success with the research of others. And, Chesborough warns, there is a legion of other, even newer companies waiting to supplant these firms, should the opportunity arise. Likewise, the TRAIL Living Lab adopts the open innovation concept by seeking new ways to collaborate with the end user, stakeholders and the business environment. As business becomes horizontal, global and networked, there is a realization, as evidenced by Chesborough's findings, that one company cannot do it alone. They must collaborate in the new borderless ecosystem of the digital age. It is argued that the innovation challenge of how best to fuse appropriate ICT with mounting age-related healthcare, could benefit from an open and user innovation model such as Living Labs.

The TRAIL Living Lab

The mission of TRAIL is to study the unmet needs of ageing citizens in rural locations in the region of the North of Ireland. The objective of TRAIL is to conduct community-facilitated and user-driven methodologies that create service and product innovations that will enable rural and ageing citizens to live independently in the heart of their communities. TRAIL will develop pilot products and services for this sector of the community, with the added benefit of validating and fine-tuning the innovation methods. Importantly, TRAIL will support a fusion of innovation models, technology and integrated community care-based approaches. This will be achieved through executing on the following development strategy components:

- Identification and prioritization of user needs;
- Developing integrated HWO demonstration models;
- Building capability through development, innovation, awareness and continuous process improvement;
- Growing the laboratory's reach and impact through geographic expansion, service intensification, advocacy and innovation based on evidence;
- Developing a sustainable business model for continued growth; and
- Conducting exploratory, evaluative and comparative empirical innovation studies that aim to understand better the Living Lab best practices, benchmarks, value chains, multi-level challenges and facilitators, and to understand better the core processes.

In the context of the European innovation system, the TRAIL model of open and user innovation links directly with the ambition of ENOLL, namely, to progress towards connecting the Lisbon Strategy [3] to a new and more user-driven European Innovation System. Moreover, TRAIL is equally in line with both the Lisbon Agenda and Northern Ireland regional development policy. For example, a key construct of Lisbon is "encouraging knowledge and innovation, by promoting more investment in research and development, by facilitating innovation, the take-up of information and communication technologies (ICT) and the sustainable use of resources, and by helping to create a strong European industrial base" – this is intrinsically linked to the social inclusion and economic growth in Northern Ireland. The Regional Development Strategy for Northern Ireland entitled "Think Create Innovate" [2] highlights the importance of a coherent innovation infrastructure; the use of innovation by the business sector; developing a culture of innovation and enterprise; and sustaining the regional innovation system as its key constructs. The TRAIL vision is congruent with this need and directly supports the development of innovation capacity to build a higher-value regional economy in Northern Ireland.

Citizen Involvement in the Innovation Process

There are major information asymmetries among potential user-innovators because much information used by product or service providers is costly to transfer or "sticky" [4]. The "stickiness" of a given unit of information is defined as the incremental expenditure required for transferring that unit from one place to another in a form usable by a specified information seeker (see von Hippel [6] for full discussion). Also, users typically do not know exactly what they want at the start of the design process. There is simply too much to know about the setting in which a novel product or service will be used for this to be possible.

Unsurprisingly, innovations developed by users are widely distributed among many users rather than concentrated among a few highly innovative firms or individuals [8]. Hence, co-operation among users and key stakeholders including firms, community, academia and research institutions, and government agencies and cities etc, are key drivers of the LL model.

Users are seen as key directors and collaborators in the process and will be involved in making comments on the performance, reliability, usefulness, safety factors, suitability or desirability of the developed concepts. In the healthcare setting, users include:

- Core Users (the priority target group): Users are older people, particularly rural dwelling, who require assistance with performing certain daily life activities and who may benefit from use of the developed service in terms of greater autonomy and quality of life (e.g. keeping in contact with family and friends, participating in activities they enjoy, enhancing feelings of safety).

- Supporting Users (who support the priority target group): these are informal or professional HWO carers who support and provide care for the user, and will be responsible for using the concepts in concert with the core users.

User engagement and eliciting user requirements is core to TRAIL operations. The purpose of a robust user requirement methodology is to secure accurate determination of the capability, characteristic, and functionality of the products and services. Ethnographic techniques and qualitative methodologies will be developed to promote 'co-operative enquiry' to assist with product and service design and advance service model evaluation methodologies. TRAIL will analyze the factors by which an older person is affected or that affects the process of daily living, e.g., (dis-)abilities, patient characteristics, level of integration with normal society/environment, social and material contextual aspects, received support and care, unmet needs, quality of life aspects.

To enhance opportunity for social empowerment the TRAIL philosophy is that networks of users will be formed from the local community.

The TRAIL Business Model

Services offered by the TRAIL living lab will consist of new products, services businesses and technologies. These will be available to enterprises, academia, public and civic bodies and to priority target group (older people) and customers who support the needs of the priority target group (informal or professional carers). The TRAIL lab offers services that are focused on helping the community and HWO to identify unmet needs, and translate these needs in service and product innovations. Specifically, TRAIL offers a family of services to identify unmet needs and to filter and rank these needs based upon the commercial or stakeholder benefit perceived. The second set of TRAIL services is based around the development and customization of living lab methodologies for ageing and rural people in Europe. It is anticipated that there is a requirement for these services in most development economies as well as in the local economies. The third area of service provision

will focus on development of processes to transfer knowledge and technology toward market concepts and innovation.
The primary stakeholders are enterprise, academia, public and civic bodies, the priority target group (older people) and users who support the needs of the priority target group (informal or professional carers). There is direct value to users who benefit from usable and working innovations, but the recipients of the most value are those HWO stakeholders who are trying to modernize social, welfare and health care working practices and service provision. The services of TRAIL are paid for by HWOs and health service modernization facilitators (government departments, philanthropic organizations) and in the first three years it is anticipated that regional development funding will support the process until it is established.

After proving the concept in the North of Ireland, the lab anticipates further growth from a wide ranging roll-out of participative action research programmes that can be developed at low cost, as well as an increase in the occurrence of efficient user-driven activities as the concept becomes embedded in rural communities. Overall, the intention is that these programmes and activities will stimulate the market in the region and arouse strategic interests of private business organizations, not-for-profit business and other stakeholders that seek to increase the rate of modernization of practices and services.

Infrastructure and Expertise

The TRAIL laboratory is located in the University of Ulster in Northern Ireland. At this site, we have designed and built two 'smart home' type environments whose purpose is to prototype technology solutions developed as part of our research programmes. We are the research partners in two projects, called Nestling Technology and NETWELL, which together will support 40 homes for ageing people in the North of Ireland. We have the hardware and software development resources and technical staff of 15 dedicated researchers to Living Lab activities. Supporting this dedicated Living Lab team are academic staff; undergraduate multidisciplinary student teams; postgraduate multidisciplinary teams; health trusts, health professionals and HWOs; several high-tech SMEs, a network of seed investors and venture capital companies; a pool of community users and access to business services from UU Science Park and incubator structures (uutech.

co.uk & nisp.co.uk & usurp.com).

The TRAIL management team and board is responsible for the administrative and technical coordination of the Living Lab, including securing efficient operation of activities, maximizing the use of resources designated to the Living Lab and minimizing the possibility of difficulties caused by lack of clarity and unexpected events. The management team aims to establish the tools, procedures and support mechanisms required for managing:

- Resources (financial and partner efforts);
- Information and knowledge generated within the Living Lab;
- Networking with ENOLL, linkages to national and European Innovation Systems; and
- Dissemination of Best Practice and continuous improvement of innovation processes.

TRAIL has already secured close to €3M in research support to drive our user-orientated, multi-disciplinary research agenda. As such it is well-funded for its research activities and the next goal is to secure funding and grow local and international interest to evolve new products and services from knowledge and technology transfer activities. TRAIL has several key research projects that involve partners from other European regions. This includes COGKNOW (www.cogknow.eu), a major eInclusion project aimed at helping people with dementia, which involves the universities of Luleå and Ulster as Scientific and Technical coordinators, respectively. The laboratory is also a core partner in the island of Ireland Nestling Technology Programme for the development of aware homes for ageing-in-place, supported by Atlantic Philanthropies. The NETWELL INTERREG-IIIa project stimulates and supports the growth and extension of new markets for ICT, digital media, Internet and wireless-based applications and services aimed at the ageing home environment on an island of Ireland cross-border basis. TRAIL also carries out a significant body of applied research directed at improving the quality of life for citizens in UK and beyond. Much of this research focuses on pervasive healthcare technologies. Current projects include two UK knowledge transfer projects on Integrated Remote Health Monitoring Service and Biometric Identification & Tracking. Other relevant project work includes CPVS, a project funded by Intel Inc & Alzheimer's Association in USA, which is exploring the possibility of developing a cell phone-based video streaming system to provide a range of memory cues to improve the independence and quality of life for patients with the eventual goal of reducing the need for institutionalization. Finally, TRAIL has several other complimentary international networks including access to the Innovation Space programme at Arizona State University.

Methods, Tools and Processes

The user group is older people in particular, with a focus on those home dwellers that will benefit from independent living resources. TRAIL will examine the particular needs of older rural dwellers and identify their complex needs, primarily along the dimensions of age (age-related impairments) and rurality (feeling of isolation and insecurity). TRAIL will examine the current provision from healthcare services providers and specialist centers and contextualize the user needs. The data collection will use a unified methodology, employing ethnographic analysis, surveys, interviews and other appropriate techniques. The proposal will assess user needs and use the developed common methodology to compare results.

Our methodology is user-driven, to maximize the impact of this research, and exchange best practice. Peoples' experiences have to be documented, evaluated and made available to groups looking for innovative solutions that may be applied in their own localities. Joint collective learning through study trips and innovative seminars, allows for meaningful sharing of the knowledge between the partners, and also permits broadening the access to the innovative solutions to other interested groups. TRAIL will promote sustainable collaboration between public, private and voluntary service providers, which will be achieved by organizing networking and cross-jurisdiction learning and knowledge transfer opportunities. Regional and international partnerships will be developed facilitating the working together of researchers with public and private service providers. TRAIL will promote the successful development of a working process that involves the ageing rural people in the service and product development process; the successful resultant development of innovative product and service know-how; IP; and other knowledge capital results.

Organization and Governance

This Living Lab brings together the most appropriate

stakeholders, researchers and innovators in Northern Ireland to address major problems with social inclusion using value-adding and effective e-services based upon a strong business rationale. The effective balance between academic research institutes, end-user representative organizations and leading-edge technology providers presents the necessary skills and experience to successfully develop and demonstrate the activities of the Living Lab. Many of the participants are community organizations, research organizations, and several industrial participants have significant R&D departments. This provides a high level of complementarily between users' needs, academic know-how, and SMEs who are proactive in research/development and innovation.

Each participating organization has been chosen for their unique blend of knowledge and expertise in a specific area with diverse skills ranging from telecommunications and software development to end-user trials and requirements gathering. The participants will draw on the full range of expertise and experience within their respective organizations to ensure the maximum success and impact on the work of the Living Lab. The LL participants are drawn from:

- Community - The community is the rural areas in Northern Ireland and encapsulates user representative groups, the physical rural and ageing community dwellers, the circle of formal HWO and informal family and friendly carers as well as the councils, boards and other public representatives. The community partners' primary aim is to seek to identify the needs of the community, in particular the needs of those older rural people in the community. The community grouping will deliver increased understanding of needs of the community.
- Academic – A strong evidence-based research base exists through the innovation network of academic partners involved. The academic partners provide research vision, and importantly, the state of the art. The academic partners' primary aim is to seek to translate identified need into supported research programmes that generate know-how and intellectual property, and identify and extend research in innovation models that can provide new ways to translate intellectual property into sustained economic activity in Northern Ireland. The University of Ulster, Northern Ireland, has multidisciplinary research teams involved in its Living

Lab from information & communication technologies; occupational therapy; health care; social care; business and management; interface, product and service design; and clinical medicine groups.

- Business - The business grouping consists of a number of SMEs located in Northern Ireland. The SMEs view technologies for ageing and rural people as an innovation-rich new market opportunity. The SMEs acknowledge the potential for market development and associated growth but are aware of the significant risks attached. The risks can be addressed by partnering with community and academic partners to develop new products and services that address need. The business partners provide the commercial know-how and expertise to evaluate intellectual property and markets and they also provide the capabilities to develop new products and services for identified markets. The business partners' primary aim is to develop sustainable, innovative products and solutions from identified intellectual property and know-how that reflects community need. Our Living Lab delivers increased innovation networking for the companies and enables them to pool scarce resources for market analysis and new product/service/process innovations.

As is evidenced from our collaboration in Trans-national research projects, TRAIL researchers have established strong linkages across Europe and beyond that demonstrate successful national and international collaboration. The Lab is developing a clear set of intellectual property principles that it can use to minimize the risk to the stakeholders as knowledge capital is developed from the TRAIL programmes.

Future Plans

The emerging TRAIL model is different to its predecessors, such as science parks and incubators, in that, it supports a community-facilitated end user-focused innovation that takes place in real-life contexts, rather than in a traditional lab or incubator. The other additional feature is the collaborative virtual network. Hence, this model offers researchers new opportunities to study innovation from a different perspective, end user innovation that is driven by the cooperation of a community of stakeholders.

TRAIL Living Labs will primarily impact upon communities

in the region and will support an economic transition of the region to a more prosperous society by supporting the economic infrastructure of the region, stimulating new higher potential enterprise creation within the region, creating open innovation systems within the region, providing a foundation for increased investment and employment opportunities in proximity to deprived areas within the region, increased economic and academic co-operation between participants and stakeholders in the region, supporting community economic development through the development of new innovation ideas in the region, and initiating actions to develop the economic resources of the area and aimed at economic revitalization in the region. The specific contextual nature of the healthcare sector in general and the needs of the elderly in particular, will offer their own peculiarities. Previous user methodologies that have been carried out in other sectors may not be easily extrapolated. It has been suggested that further research into efficient user driven methodologies to extract rich diagnosis of user needs is warranted, including the appropriateness and adoption of the lead user method.

References

[1] Chesbrough, H. (2003) Open Innovation: The New Imperative for Creating and Profiting from Technology. Boston, MA: Harvard Business School Press.

[2] DETI, 2003, 'think|create|innovate - the Regional Innovation Strategy for Northern Ireland', Published by the Department of Enterprise, Trade and Investment, www.detini.gov.uk/thinkcreateinnovate, June 2003, Accessed 10 September 2007

[3] Lisbon Agenda, European Council special meeting, 23-24 March 2000, Lisbon, Portugal, European Parliament, http://www.europarl.europa.eu/summits/lis1_en. htm, Retrieved September 10, 2007

[4] Lüthje, C., Herstatt, C. and von Hippel. (2005) User-innovations and "local" information: The case of mountain biking. Research Policy. 34, 951-965.

[5] Niitamo, VP., Kulkki, S., Eriksson, M. & Hribernik, K.A. (2006) State-of-the-Art and Good Practice in the field of Living Labs. In 12th International Conference on Concurrent Enterprising (ICE), 26-28 June 2006. Milan, Italy: VE-Forum Platform.

[6] von Hippel, E. (1994) "Sticky information", and the Locus of Problem Solving: Implications for Innovation. Management Science. 40 (4), 429-439.

[7] von Hippel, E. & Tyre, M. (1995) How "learning by doing" is Done: Problem Identification in Novel Process Equipment. Research Policy. 24 (January), 1-12.

[8] von Hippel, E. (2005) Democratizing Innovation. Cambridge, MA: MIT Press.

Aging, Disability and Independence
W.C. Mann (Ed.)
IOS Press, 2008

doi:10.3233/978-1-58603-902-8-119

Multidisciplinary Generation of Car Design Requirements for Older Drivers: A Functional Analysis

Corinna Flöck[1], Mounib Mekhilef[1], Julie Le Cardinal[1]
[1]Department of Industrial Engineering
Ecole Centrale Paris

Abstract: The proportion of older people in the population is rising, as is the proportion of older driving licence holders. The needs and abilities of older drivers therefore need to be considered in vehicle design. Our research is focussing on the multidisciplinary identification of design requirements for aged drivers. Research on older drivers has become a field of interest in various research domains and technical areas but coherent results are still missing. We need interdisciplinary approaches directly aimed at supporting older road users. We suggest a functional analysis in order to assist us in identifying the actors, aims and limits of our system. Our analysis is motivated by the need to contrast diverse perspectives to obtain new knowledge and research directions. The functional analysis allows us to make statements about the knowledge needed by designers and the interrelation of actors and factors according to system. It also helps us to formulate further research recommendations for car design requirements for older drivers.

Keywords: Older Driver, Ageing society, Multidisciplinary Approach, Functional Analysis, Requirement Generation

Introduction

Mobility needs and safety issues of the ageing population have in the last several years become an issue of interest for research, industry and governments, especially in the industrialised world. In this context, special attention is paid to older drivers. This is due in part to the expected increase of older persons in the population. It is estimated that by 2050 one quarter or more of the population of the OECD countries will be over the age of 65.

As the proportion of older people in the population rises, the proportion of older drivers is also increasing. Owning and driving a car can play an important role in providing senior citizens access to social facilities and offer the possibility to live an active and independent life. Independent out-of-home mobility is an important aspect of older persons' well-being. Previous research has shown that mobility and the ability to leave the home are among the essential aspects in the quality of life of older persons. This paper is based on the need for the identification of design requirements, responding to the specific needs of older drivers and includes a functional analysis of these needs.

Objectives

Our analysis is motivated by the need to contrast diverse perspectives that will lead to formulating coherent design requirements for older drivers. The results will then enable Design Engineers to include the particular needs of the older generation into their design processes and adapt vehicles according to these needs. The functional analysis proposed in this article, is a first step towards this aim and will help in formulating further research recommendations for car design requirements for older drivers.

Evolution of the research field

Research on older drivers is a relatively new topic of interest although some general interest was expressed as early as the 1930s. A first important wave of research on older drivers took place at the end of the 1960s, mainly in the US. This research was influenced by Thomas W. Planek who published several articles and books, addressing the effects of ageing on driving performance. He considers older drivers as over age 55, but he states that certain impairments, which could influence driving, could be present as early as age 50. His main research interest was to identify deficits and impairments of ageing persons in relationship to driving [6] [7]. At this time the question of ageing and driving received little attention in Europe. Some age-related controls or restrictions concerning driving licensing were introduced, but this topic didn't raise any common interest at governmental and research institutions [1].

A report published by the Organisation for Economic Co-Operation and Development (OECD) in 1985, addressing safety of older road users and current research, encouraged widespread interest among researchers and governments. The report did not focus on older drivers, but approached the topic more from a generic point of view and discussed issues of older road users in general. It discussed older persons as unprotected road users, reporting that they were over-represented in fatal traffic accidents. The report also discussed the use of alternative travel options [5].

In the US the focus of research at this time was on private

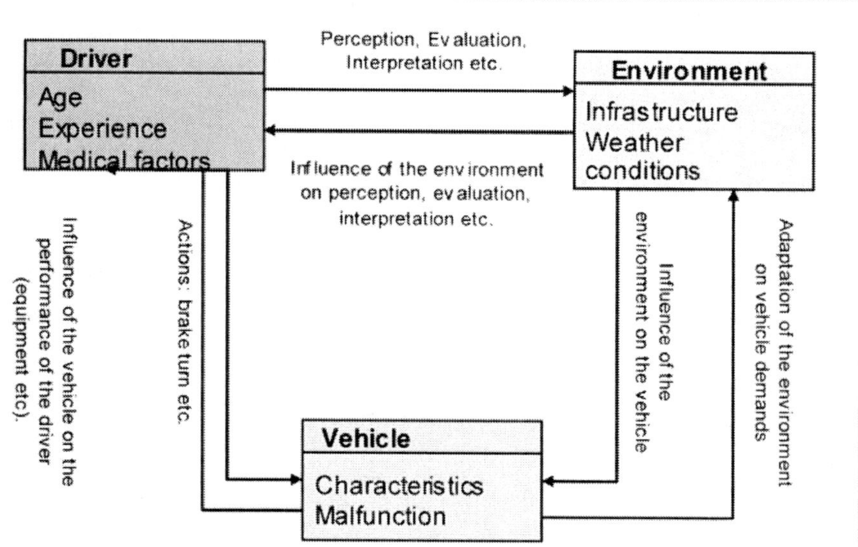

Figure 1: The Driver Vehicle Environment System

car use. This is related in part to the fact that, in the US, more people lived in suburban areas where a car was essential for daily activities. Since this time interest in issues related to older drivers increased not only in Europe and North America, but also in Australia and some Asian countries. Today investigators from a number of scientific fields and technical areas are addressing older driver issues, and the topic is raised at many international conferences.

Method

To create competitive advantages, the automotive industry must address user needs. A holistic, multi-disciplinary approach combining perspectives from various fields and research domains was used to identify issues that relate to older drivers. A functional analysis acts as a support mechanism for mastering the complexity and interrelations in the field. Based on the demographic changes and changing user needs, the present research follows an innovative approach for the product development process and assists in defining requirements for car designers to address the specific needs of older drivers.

Functional analyses are often used to define specific needs and requirements in new product development. The functional analysis approach takes into consideration the various points of view of different research domains including the environmental aspects influencing older drivers. Typically, functional analyses are conducted by multi-disciplinary teams. Functional analyses encourage innovation within a company and help establish a common view on a new product or service and the identification of previously neglected opportunities.

The functional analysis is based on "value engineering" which originated at General Electric during World War II. Because of the war, there were shortages of skilled labour, raw materials, and component parts. These shortages led Lawrence Miles and Harry Erlicher at General Electric Co. to look for acceptable substitutes. They noticed that these substitutions often reduced costs, improved the product, or both. What started out as an accident of necessity turned into a systematic process. They called their technique "value analysis"[3]. Since then the method has been used in research and industry and has been adapted and readjusted in numerous ways. We base our approach on the methodology called SWING that has been proposed by the French company COVALENCE and which focuses on the identification of key functions related to our system.

A functional analysis also helps to gain a clear picture about the usability of a product or a service, and assists in identifying main actors in the field. In our case, we use the functional analysis as a step towards the development of multi-disciplinary design requirements for older drivers, which in turn will be used by car designers for the development of future cars. Knowledge about older drivers and their needs is available, but a common understanding, helping the designer to adapt vehicles is still missing. Our analysis is based upon the Driver-Vehicle-Environment (DVE) Model. According to Miller's definition of a living system [4], we define the DVE as an open and living system since each component (i.e. driver, vehicle, infrastructure, traffic, etc.) is constantly interacting with its environment by means of information and matter-energy exchanges. We consider not only the driver, but the whole interaction between the driver, the vehicle and the environment in which the driver is acting, thus assuring consideration of the whole system. The DVE is a well established model, used in various research domains, including transportation research and accidentology. It addresses three main points of view and assures a systemic view. It is enriched by the perspectives of several disciplines and research domains and the analysis of methodologies to gather knowledge and information.

The functional analysis aims at the formulation of functions, describing the optimum behaviour of the system and its terms of usability. It also helps to analyse cost efficiency and resources needed to determine a service or a product.

The Functional Analysis

The SWING method of functional analysis introduces a formalised approach, leading to well structured results that are described in the following paragraphs. The functional analysis consists of 4 main steps:

- General analysis of the system
- Identification of the system's environments
- Formulation of functions
- Validation of functions

General Analysis

Before formulating the functions and identifying possible environments it is important to begin with a general analysis to form a first impression about the system itself, its application areas, and limits. We therefore use the visualisation of the "horned animal" as introduced in the SWING method and its formalism represented in Figure 2.

This validity control aims at the determination of:

- The main user
- The cause of the study (why?),
- Which objectives it aims at (for what?), in order determine the necessity to conduct the study.

Figure 3 shows the model of the horned animal projected in our case.

A fourth question not represented in the graphical representation is "What are the risks of evolution or disappearance of the system." In our case possible scenarios would include:

- Sharp decline in number of older persons
- Driving licensing restrictions, for people over a certain age
- Complete and inclusive knowledge about Design requirements for older drivers, making further development unnecessary

The identification of environments

A second step is the identification of environments that act with the system. The so called "octopus" is important in to describe the elements of the subject's environment, the transfer functions (FT) between two elements by the mean of the subject, and the constraint functions (FC) which the subject has to respect for an element of environment. At this stage it is important to be as inclusive as possible, to ensure that crucial aspects are not neglected during the next steps of the functional analysis. The beneficiary entity is thus identified; the subject and objective of the study are formalized. In our case we identified the following main environments.

Reasons for the clustering

To present environments in a comprehensive way, we propose to use clusters and sub clusters. Clusters represent the main elements identified as having influence on the process. Sub clusters are built whenever specifications are seen as necessary and only apply in cases where a difference in outcome towards the system to be analysed occurs.

The DVE System as presented in Figure 1 is a well established model used in various domains, such as transportation research

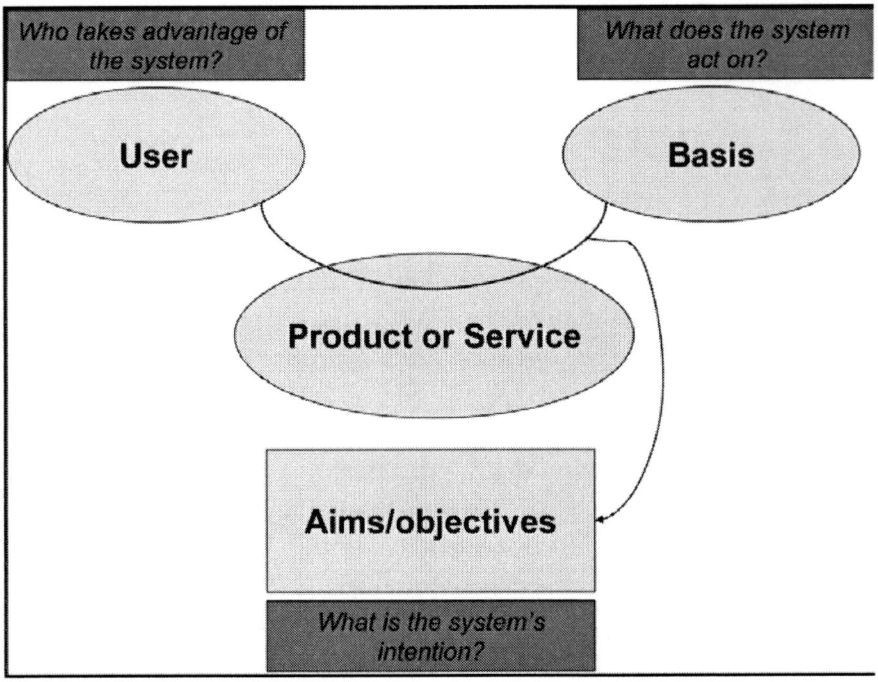

Figure 2: The Horned Animal

and traffic psychology. It covers the three main points of view and assures a systemic view. It is thus a logical step to consider these 3 elements as large clusters of environments in the functional analysis. One cluster is represented by the "vehicle", which we mainly break down according to primary, secondary and tertiary safety systems and their functionalities. Also the "environment" is considered as one cluster. Here we summarise mainly aspects related to regulations, road infrastructure and weather conditions. The driver himself plays a particular role in this case and is also considered an environment. The older driver is the heart of this functional analysis and all information provided and used is meant to support the driver. The driver acts as an expert from his/her own particular point of view and is consulted in the process to assure end-user acceptance and usability of the proposed solutions.

Ageing is associated with increased incidence of physical and cognitive impairments. As health conditions and cognitive abilities have a major influence on driving, we suggest a cluster "health conditions", which addresses cognitive and physical impairments. This is not a sub-cluster of the driver, as it is a major element that must be addressed when considering design requirements for older drivers.

Another environment relates to the many "experts" (e.g.

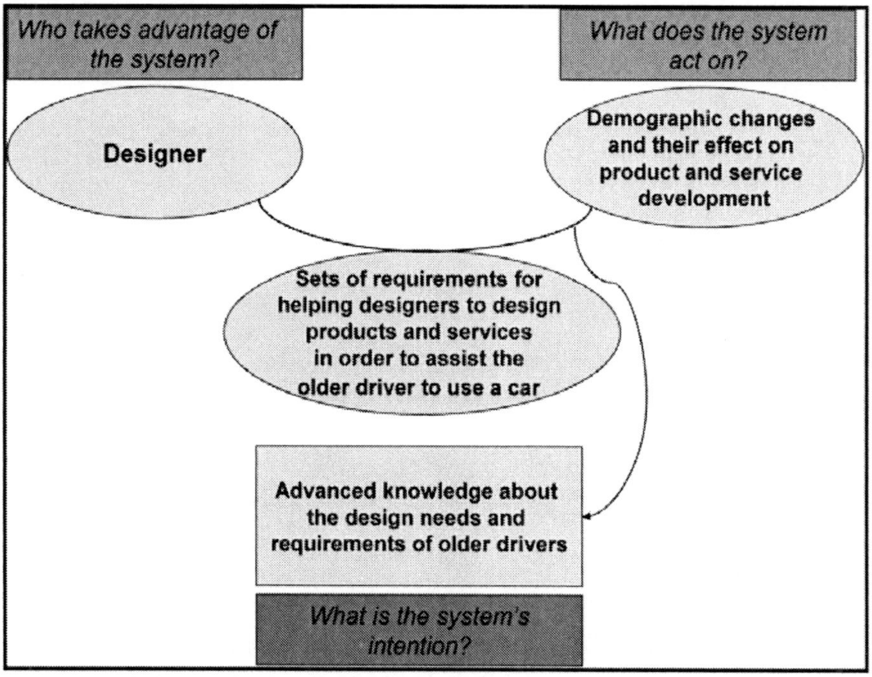

Figure 3: The Horned Animal According to Our System

Psychologist, Physician,), as they provide important knowledge for the identification of design requirements from several points of view. We see "experts" as crucial, as the aim of the overall study is having a clear picture about the design needs of older drivers and a coherent set of requirements combing various viewpoints.

"Designers" can of course be seen as one element of the 'experts' cluster, as they can provide their input and point of view during the process. Nevertheless we represent them in a separate group, as they will act as an end-user of the developed solutions and thus intervene at a different level during the process.

A sixth large cluster is built around the different kinds of "knowledge" and their sources. We consider several sources of information. Mainly we base our research on story telling by the experts, and the analysis of existing databases, like the EDA.

Formulation of functions

Out of 113 transfer functions and 33 constraint functions that have been identified through the establishment of relations between the outlined environments shown in Figure 3, we have chosen the following key functions to be considered for further analysis. They represent main aspects of the system and will help us to determine additional factors.

FC32: The system should consider the effect of driving under different weather conditions

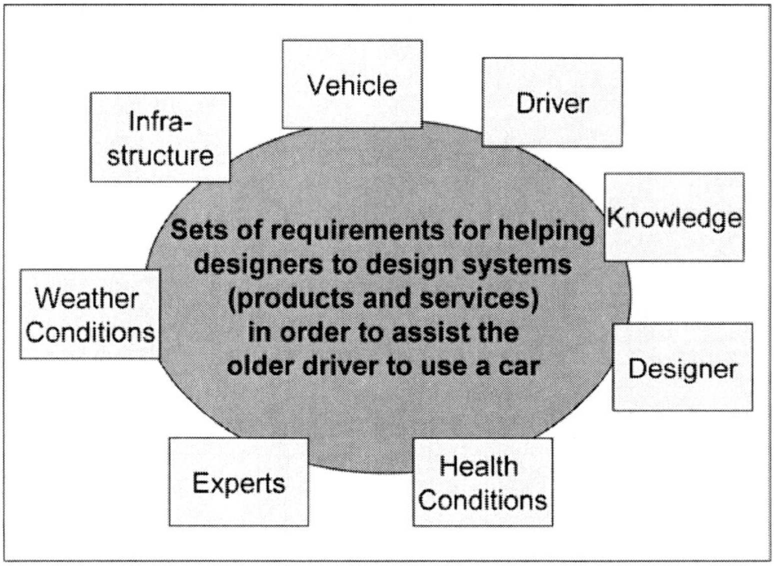

Figure 4: Main environments related to the topic

FC33: The system should consider the influence of health problems on driving
FC29: The system should be described to be usable by car designers
FC25: The system should be able to limit accidents
FT113: The system should give inclusive information to car designers concerning the influence of environmental circumstances on older drivers
FT49: The system should enable car designers to design cars based on multi-disciplinary expert knowledge
F26: The system should give information to car designers about the effect of visual impairments on the perception of intersections
FT8: The system should give information to car manufacturers concerning different health conditions and their implications on driving
FT6: The system should enable embedded system designers to provide new systems for car designers

Validation of the functions

After having identified these key functions, we characterise them by responding to the questions concerning the system. In this case we use them to validate the functions. This means that we proof the usefulness of the proposed function to be sure

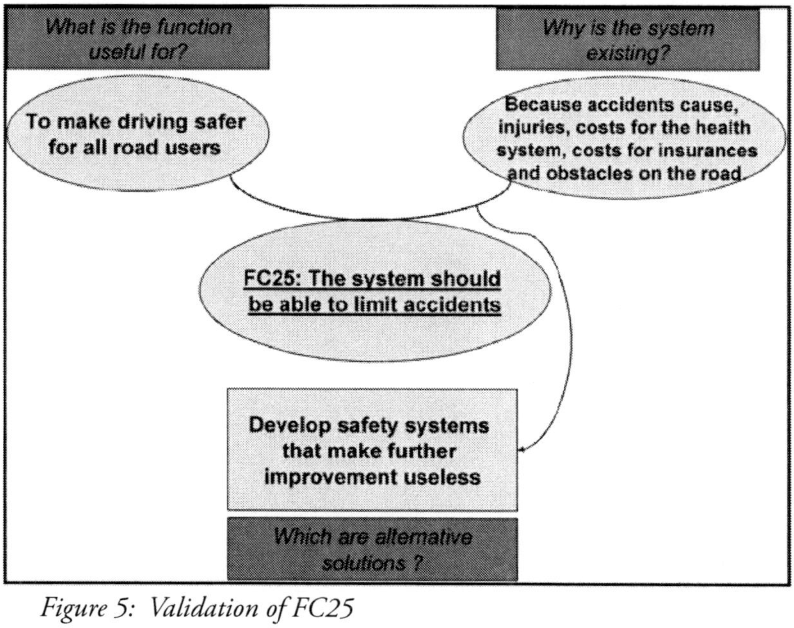

Figure 5: Validation of FC25

that we can use it for further analysis. We call this methodology ABAC, which stands for the French "Analyse des Buts, des Alternatives et des Causes" – Analysis of Aims, Alternatives and Reasons. In general it can be stated that a function is validated if an answer to all questions can be provided. The answer can either be given through new aspects and knowledge or through another function and is represented in the following way.

- Buts/ Aims: What is the function useful for?
- Alternatives: For a specific aim what are alternative solutions to achieve them?
- Causes/ Reasons: What are the reasons for the system's existence?
- For what reasons might the system become useless or disappear?

Here are two examples for the validation of functions. For graphical representation we use again the "horned animal".

<u>FC25: The system should be able to limit accidents</u>
B1: To make driving safer for all road users
B2: To avoid costs due to accidents
B3: To avoid people getting injured or killed
B4: To make driving safer for older drivers

A1: develop safety systems that make further improvement useless.
A2: find a solution that makes accidents "less expensive"
A3: primary and secondary safety systems get developed

C1: Because accidents cause, injuries, result in health related and insurance, and result in obstacles on the road, their reduction is a main aim.
C2b: primary and secondary safety systems are able to avoid any kind of accident.

<u>FC32: The system should consider the effect of driving under different weather conditions</u>
B1: To enable car designers to consider these effects during the product development phase
B2: To gain knowledge about the cause of accidents and avoid

them in the future through new embedded systems based on this knowledge

A1: Designers collect information themselves. Designers consider that this information is not relevant and ignore it.
A2: accident causation and avoidance are not treated under consideration of climate

C1: Because the different weather conditions have an influence on the driving performance of older persons and should be considered when defining sets of requirements, to enhance safety.
Cb2: Cars become so smart that they automatically adapt to weather conditions.

Conclusion

The functional analysis shows that the design to support older drivers' safe mobility, should take into account the special characteristics of older persons, both in terms of the different facets of the ageing process and in terms of the older persons' mobility needs. In addition, the design should also capture the heterogeneity of the older population. Those categorized as "elderly" vary greatly in terms of their chronological age, functionality, socio-economical status, gender, and travel patterns. The needs and abilities of older drivers must be considered in vehicle design. Our research is focussing on the multidisciplinary identification of design requirements for aged drivers. Research on older drivers has become a field of interest in various research domains and technical areas but coherent results are still missing. We need interdisciplinary approaches directly aiming at supporting older road users.

Our analysis has shown us that most functions are based on the assessment of the behaviour of the older driver. We therefore assume that particular attention should be paid to the consideration of the point of view of older drivers themselves. We suggest a user-centred approach for product development and a systemic analysis of the field according to the epistemological approach proposed by Piaget [8] and further extended by Le Moigne [2]. We are now able to describe the research field from a systemic point of view, which makes it possible to identify key elements and to formulate coherent research questions for future studies in the field of older drivers

The functional analysis provides an overall picture of the key elements, stakeholders and decision makers in research of older drivers. It offers insights into the complex system, shows interrelations, and can guide multidisciplinary research on requirements to be considered by car designers and manufacturers. We suggest a systemic approach for further research activities in the field, to obtain detailed and comparable results stemming from different sources. It is evident that the development of design requirements for older drivers is a complex task, requiring consideration of many factors of influence.

References

[1] Hakamies-Blomqvist L. and Henriksson P. (1999). Cohort effects in older drivers' accident type distribution: are older drivers as old as they used to be? Transportation Research Part F: Traffic Psychology and Behaviour, 2(3) 131-138.

[2] Le Moigne J.L. (1990). La modélisation des systèmes complexes, Paris. Dunod.

[3] Miles, L. (1971). Techniques of Value Analysis and Engineering. McGraw-Hill.

[4] Miller J.G. (1995). Living Systems. University Press of Colorado.

[5] OECD (2001). Organisation for Economic Co-operation and Development: Ageing and Transport: Mobility Needs and Safety Issues, Paris.

[6] Planek T.W. (1972). The aging driver in today's traffic: a critical review. In Planek T.W., Mann W.A. and Wiener E.L. (Eds.). Aging and highway safety: the elderly in a mobile society. Chapel Hill, N. C.: Highway Safety Research Center.

[7] Planek T. and Overland R. (1973). How Aging Affects the Driver. Traffic Safety, 73(2)

[8] Piaget, J. (1975). L'équilibration des structures cognitives, problème central du dévélopment. P.U.F., Paris.

[9] http://wendt.library.wisc.edu/miles/refcenter.html

Aging, Disability and Independence
W.C. Mann (Ed.)
IOS Press, 2008

doi:10.3233/978-1-58603-902-8-131

Accommodations for Mobility In The Workplace: A Comparison of Workers with And Without Wheeled Mobility Devices

Jesse S Zolna, MS; Dory Sabata OTD, OTR/L;
and Jon Sanford, M.Arch.
Georgia Institute of Technology, Ctr. for
Assistive Technology & Environmental Access

Abstract: Modifications to personal workstations and architectural changes to the work environment are some of the most common types of accommodation used to facilitate work performance by people with mobility impairments (Zolna, Sanford, Sabata, & Goldthwaite, in press). However, workplace accommodations may vary by what mobility function the person finds to be difficult. For instance, one might modify a personal workstation to reach their desk or equipment, but a different kind of accommodation to a personal workstation could be used to improve seating for those remaining at the desk or using a computer for long periods of time.

Moreover, those who use a wheelchair may use different types of accommodations than those who are ambulatory. For example, architectural changes made to mitigate environmental barriers such as getting up stairs might be different to accommodate a person in a wheelchair than to accommodate an ambulatory person with balance or vision problems. Therefore, research regarding workplace accommodations for people with mobility impairments should examine the specific functional limitation(s) addressed by the accommodation.

Background

The workplace can be a challenging environment for people with mobility limitations. Mobility impairments of various types, such as spinal-cord injury, arthritis, age-related musculoskeletal disorders, amputation, repetitive strain injuries, and multiple sclerosis lead to functional limitations that impede performance of tasks necessary for work. The Accessibility Guidelines put forth by the Americans with Disabilities Act were designed to improve access for people with disabilities to public spaces including the workplace. However, achieving these goals involves more than just improving access to the work facility. Workplace accommodations are also provided to people with mobility impairments to mitigate functional limitations and facilitate successful work performance.

Among the goals of providing workplace accommodations is increasing the participation of people with disabilities in the workforce, improving the chances that people return to work after injury (Tomassen, Post, & van Asbeck, 2000), and reducing health related job loss [1].

The severity of physical limitation impeding mobility is negatively associated with gainful employment [5] [16] and when studying the provision of broad accommodation categories, differences in the limitations addressed by a similar accommodation might be overlooked. To better understand workplace accommodations for people with mobility impairments, research must avoid blending different kinds of mobility limitations into one general category. Using a more precise description of what a person with a mobility impairment can and cannot do in the workplace might help better understand how accommodations facilitate work performance.

The International Classification of Functioning, Disability and Health (ICF) provides a taxonomy of functional limitations related to mobility impairments and general work tasks that might offer a more precise picture of impairment than a broad, general category of mobility limitation. According to the IFC's classification, there are four general types of mobility limitation: (1) changing and maintaining body position, (2) carrying, moving and handling objects, (3) walking and moving, and (4) moving around using transportation (WHO, 2001).

Much of the workstation accommodations literature addresses a general category of accommodation that includes any ergonomic improvement to a workstation or any changes made to office furnishing [3] [8] [14][23]. Workplace accommodations for people who have mobility limitations are likely to vary greatly depending on whether or not they use a mobility device (such as a wheelchair) on a regular basis. That is, people who use a wheelchair have difficulty working at a standard desk, leading to functional limitations associated with sitting in a chair, a lack of workspace, and getting up from their desk [15]. For people with mobility impairments who do not use a wheelchair, functional limitations are often related to activities that can not be done by people in wheelchairs, such as having to stand on a hard surface or repeatedly bend over to complete a task [12]. As a result of the differences in limitations, the workstation accommodations provided might actually be very different. In addition, the appropriate accommodation might be usable by other employees.

Most literature addressing workplace accommodations for people with mobility limitations focuses on either workers who use a mobility device or workers who do not use a mobility device. This literature often does not provide much in the way of examples of specific modification types [3] [8] [11] [13] [14] [20] [23]. The types of accommodations used by these two groups are likely to vary even though mobility remains the issue for both of these groups. This is because tasks that are difficult for people with mobility impairments are strongly associated with the use of a mobility device. Moreover, the degree of use for common accommodations by people with mobility impairments who use wheeled mobility devices, and others with mobility impairments who do not use mobility devices has not been clearly documented in the literature.

In the present study, researchers were interested in identifying the types of accommodations used to address difficulties with mobility, specifically comparing those who use wheeled mobility devices with those who do not.

Methods

A sample of 244 respondents with self-reported mobility limitations and a history of employment were included in this study. Mobility limitations were indicated by difficulty with one or more of the following: keeping their body in position, changing position, moving around, or manipulating objects. Additionally respondents were divided into two groups. One group included those who used wheeled mobility devices and the other group consisted of those who did not use wheeled mobility devices for their mobility difficulties.

Participants were recruited through a number of methods. The first method used was a mass mailing to households that were known to have at least one person with a disability. Additional recruitment efforts were targeted through listservs and disability-specific organizations. Further, an open invitation to complete the survey was posted on the research center's website.

The survey included questions regarding: 1) demographics, including age, gender, income and education of workers with disabilities; 2) prevalence of mobility limitations that affect workers' abilities and 3) types of accommodations used for these mobility difficulties. Finally, respondents were asked to indicate whether their accommodations were used only by themselves or by others as well.

The survey was administered to the respondents in three different ways: online survey (79% of the total), mailed survey (20% of total), and telephone interviews (less than 1% of the total). Online responses were the preferred method of administering the survey, while the mailed and telephone versions were provided to individuals who requested them.

Survey data were analyzed with SPSS v13. To assess differences between the accommodations used by the wheeled mobility group and the others with mobility difficulties, we performed two-tailed independent sample t-tests. If Levene's test for equality of variances was significant, equal variances were not assumed. An alpha level of $p < .05$ was used in all t-tests.

Results

Of the 224 respondents, 114 indicated using a wheeled mobility device (either a wheelchair, power wheelchair, or scooter) on a daily basis. One hundred ten participants did not use any type of wheeled mobility device on a daily basis. However, this group did include 11 respondents who used a walker and 37 who used a cane. Some of these mobility limitations might have been due to vision limitations, since 52 of the 110 in this group reported an additional functional limitation related to vision and 84 reported use of glasses.

For the two groups of participants in this study workplace accommodations were considered in terms of four specific mobility tasks and the frequency of different types of workplace accommodations used for each of those tasks are outlined in Table 1. When comparing the types of accommodations used by persons both with and without wheeled mobility devices, several mobility tasks were considered. First, accommodations used for positioning, including both keeping and changing positions, were compared across the two groups of study participants. Those without wheeled mobility devices were significantly more likely to have an ergonomic/custom designed workstation to better position the work to alleviate difficulties keeping their body in position, $t = 2.207$ (2, 212), $p = .029$. This group was also significantly more likely to indicate that they received no accommodation to alleviate difficulties changing positions during work, $t = 2.187$ (2, 207), $p = .030$. In comparison, those with wheeled mobility devices were

Table 1.

Abilities that are needed to do your current or most recent job and related difficulties	Accommodations that were made to diminish difficulties at work	% of users with mobility device	% of users without mobility device
Keeping your body in position (i.e. staying in positions to perform tasks)	**None**	-	-
	Ergonomic/custom workstation	18	30*
	Ergonomic/custom designed chairs	18	13
	Steps or lifts	11	17
Changing positions (i.e. moving from one position to another)	**None**	-	-
	Ergonomic/custom workstation	27*	9
	Ergonomic/custom designed chairs	8	11
	Steps or lifts	8	5
	Back support belt	2	5
Moving around (i.e. moving across spaces)	**None**	-	-
	Accessible transportation	47*	26
	Restroom modification(s)	43*	8
	Accessible parking	38*	15
	Ramps	33	11
	Automatic door	33*	10
	Flexible work schedule	27*	19
	Use of a wheelchair or scooter (at work only)	24*	5
	Elevator	25	22
	Hand rails	13	12
	Emergency call button	28*	9
Manipulating objects (e.g. grasping, turning, lifting, or moving objects)	None	19	16
	Personal assistant	14	10
	Buddy system	15	14
	Modifications made to equipment or machinery	14*	4
	Gripping aids	11	8
	Carts	4	13*
	Clamping devices to hold materials	6*	1
	Job task redesign	6	5

* $p < 0.05$

more likely to receive an ergonomic/custom designed workstation to better position the work and alleviate difficulties changing positions during work, $t = 3.613$ (2, 194), $p < .001$.

Next, this study considered the types of accommodations used by people with and without mobility devices for addressing difficulties moving around. To mitigate difficulties moving around, t-tests showed that people who use a wheeled mobility device were significantly more likely to report using accessible transportation, $t = 3.326$ (2, 220), $p = .001$, accessible parking, $t = 4.084$ (2, 207), $p > .001$, ramps, $t = 4.194$ (2, 197), $p > .001$, restroom modifications, $t = 6.510$ (2, 178), $p > .001$, automatic doors, t

= 4.416 (2, 193), $p > .001$, use of a wheelchair at work only, $t = 4.004$ (2, 174), $p > .001$, and emergency call buttons, $t = 3.762$ (2, 193), $p > .001$.

In comparing the types of accommodations used by these two groups for manipulating objects, the group with wheeled mobility devices was significantly more likely to report modifications to equipment or machinery, $t = 2.790$ (2, 175), $p = .001$, and the use of clamping devices to hold materials, $t = 2.149$ (2, 149), $p = .033$. Alternatively, those without wheeled mobility devices were more likely to use carts as an accommodation for manipulating objects, $t = 2.539$ (2, 168), $p = .012$.

In comparing whether accommodations were universally designed or not, those in the no mobility device group were significantly more likely to report that their accommodation was intended to be used only by them, but was used by others as well $t = 3.531$(2, 222), $p < .001$, while those in the mobility device group were significantly more likely to report that their primary accommodation was intended to be used by others, but was only used by them $t = 2.506$(2, 222), $p = .013$.

Table 1.

Discussion

Both workers with and without wheeled mobility devices reported using ergonomic workstations and chairs as common accommodations for positioning. However they used these accommodations for different types of tasks relative to positioning. Those with mobility devices used ergonomic workstations to address difficulties with changing positions, while those without mobility devices used these accommodations for maintaining body position at work.

Modifying personal work stations.

The results reported here suggest that difficulties keeping position and changing position at work are often mitigated by the provision of ergonomic workstations. Adjustable height workstations are important to work for people with mobility impairments [13] and modular office furniture is an important way to provide ergonomic workstations [21]. Examples include changes to desks, modified workspace layout [18], bringing frequently used items closer, lowering work surfaces, raising the height of the desk, rearranging furniture and desk items, or using adjustable tables and shelves [21]. Computer access and the provisions of input controls for computer access [13] and computer keyboards to alter the positioning of the user are also important workstation design features for accommodating people with mobility impairments [10].

The results of this survey suggest that people who have a mobility device (such as a wheelchair) use ergonomic workstation accommodations to alleviate difficulties changing positions during work, while people who have a mobility impairment but do not use a mobility device use ergonomic workstation accommodations to alleviate difficulties keeping position during work. It is important to understand how employees with different types of mobility limitations and functional impairments will use similar accommodations to further understand what accommodations will be successful in a certain situation. Based on the functional limitations of the user, the modification of a workstation for people with different mobility impairments can have widely different benefits and results. For example, the use of a wheelchair is generally not seen as a barrier to operating a computer while functional impairments related to fine movements are seen as a barrier [3]. The results of this survey also suggest that people with wheelchairs are more likely to get modifications to equipment or machinery and clamps, both of which can be similar to ergonomic improvements to workstations, to help them manipulate objects. Further research is needed to understand which types of workstation modifications are most appropriate for each limitation and mobility group and to better understand how different types of modifications address each limitation.

Architectural changes. Among this sample of people with mobility limitations difficulties with moving through space appear to be best mitigated by architectural accommodations. People with all types of mobility impairments are likely to have functional limitations that lead to problems moving through space, such as fatigue, pain, physical weakness, an inability to stand for long periods or [2] [9] [21], environmental barriers to transportation such as parking [5] and commuting [15], or trouble accessing spaces including bathrooms [7], break rooms (Scherer, 1988), and kitchens [9] [15]. Appropriate accommodations help people with mobility limitations climb stairs, walk long distances, or use doors and gates [6]. Examples of accommodations found in the literature include ramps, elevators, parking [23], floor surface changes, environmental control, signage, evacuation routes [4], low wattage overhead lights task lighting [18], and adjustments to entrances[14]. However, most of the research examining the provisions of architectural accommodations combines all these separate types of accommodations into one general group. The results of this study show that accommodations provided to reduce difficulties moving through space are much more common for people with wheelchairs than for people without wheelchairs. This is the case for many individual accommodation types included in our survey and suggests that there is a clear difference between people with and without mobility devices in the need for accommodations addressing moving through space. However, the types of accommodations were similar and all types were used by both groups.

Those in the mobility device group were significantly more likely to report that their accommodation was intended to be used by others as well as themselves, while those in the no mobility device group were significantly more likely to report that their primary accommodation was not intended to be used by others. This might reflect the fact that employees who use a mobility device are also more likely to view architectural accommodations as intended to help them move through space. However, people who do not use a mobility device are likely to consider an architectural accommodation usable by everyone including themselves. In addition, many accommodations used to help people with mobility impairments can be directly attributed to a person with a mobility device, but people without a mobility device will use the accommodation without considering the accommodation as their own. It is likely that these architectural accommodations are a natural fit for Universal Design. However, given that people who do use a mobility device use the same general types of accommodations, it might make sense for the goals of Universal Design to more explicitly include guidelines that aid people who use a mobility device.

Conclusions

Modifying a workstation often involves applying ergonomic principles to redesign work and workspaces. It is important to realize that providing ergonomic workstations as accommodations for people with mobility impairments must address more than just strength requirements to reduce the physical demand of work on employees [21]. While ergonomic workstations can be used to reduce the physical demands of work tasks, these accommodations can also address the positioning of people with mobility impairments so that they may perform their job tasks [8]. Accommodations for employees who have mobility impairments should consider redesign of work and workspaces to mitigate physical demands related to particular functional limitations.

Employees who use a mobility device more often receive an ergonomic workstation accommodation to help them change positions during work while employees with mobility limitations who do not use a mobility device commonly receive an ergonomic workstation accommodation to alleviate difficulties with keeping their positions during work. The present data suggests that employees who use a mobility device such as a wheelchair or scooter receive the same general accommodation type for very different reasons than those who are not wheeled mobility users. This could have implications for the type of ergonomic workstation provided to an employee with disabilities. Further research should explore the differences and similarities between these workstation accommodations and the implications for universal design.

References

[1] Allaire, S. H., Li, W., & LaValley, M. P. (2003). Work Barriers Experienced and Job Accommodations Used by Persons with Arthritis and other Rheumatic Diseases. Rehabilitation Counseling Bulletin, 46(3), 147-156.

[2] Beveridge, S., Craddock, S. H., Liesener, J., Stapleton, M., & Hershenson, D. (2002). Income: A Framework for Conceptualizing the Career Development of Persons with Disabilities. Rehabilitation Counseling Bulletin, 45(4).

[3] Bruyère , S., Erickson, E., & VanLooy, S. (2005). Information Technology and the Workplace: Implications for Persons with Disabilities: Implications for persons with disabilities. Disability Studies Quarterly, 25(2).

[4] Butterfield, T. M., & Ramseur, J. H. (2004). Research and case study findings in the area of workplace accommodations including provisions for assistive technology: A literature review. Technology and Disability, 16(4), 201-210.

[5] Chapin, M. H., & Kewman, D. G. (2001). Factors affecting employment following spinal cord injury: A qualitative study. Rehabilitation Psychology, 46(4), 400-416.

[6] Conroy, L., & McKenna, K. (1999). Vocational outcome following spinal cord injury. Spinal Cord, 37(9), 624-633.

[7] Cornell, P. o. E. a. D. (2000). Workplace Accommodations for Persons with Musculoskeletal Disorders. Ithaca: Program on Employment and Disability, Cornell University.

[8] deJonge, D. M., & Rodger, S. A. (2006). Consumer identified barriers and strategies for optimising technology use in the workplace. Disability and Rehabilitation: Assistive Technology, 1(1-2), 79-88.

[9] Dowler, D. L., Hirsh, A. E., Kittle, R. D., & Hendricks, D. J. (1996). Outcomes of reasonable accommodations in the workplace. Technology and Disability, 5, 345-354.

[10] Fagarasanu, M., & Kumar, S. (2003). Carpal tunnel syndrome due to keyboarding and mouse tasks: a review. International Journal of Industrial Ergonomics, 31(2), 119-136.

[11] Hedrick, B., Pape, T. L.-B., Heinemann, A. W., Ruddell, J. L., & Reis, J. (2006). Employment issues and assitive technology use for persons with spinal cord injury. Journal of Rehabilitation Research and Development, 43(2), 185-198.

[12] Inge, K. J., Strobel, W., Wehman, P., Todd, J., & P. Targett. (2000). Vocational outcomes for persons with severe physical disabilities: Design and implementation of workplace supports. NeuroRehabilitation, 15(3), 175-187.

[13] LoPresti, E. F., Brienza, D. M., & Angelo, J. (2002). Head-operated computer controls: effect of control method on performance for subjects with and without disability. Interacting with Computers, 14(4), 359-377.

[14] McNeal, D. R., Somerville, N. J., & Wilson, D. J. (1999). Work problems and accommodations reported by persons who are postpolio or have a spinal cord injury. Assistive Technology, 11(2), 137-157.

Aging, Disability and Independence
W.C. Mann (Ed.)
IOS Press, 2008

doi:10.3233/978-1-58603-902-8-141

Aging Educators with Disabilities: Experiences with Accommodations

Karen Milchus, MS, ATP
Center for Assistive Technology and Environmental Access, Georgia Tech.

Abstract: Science, technology, engineering and math (STEM) educators aging with or into disability may need accommodations in order to teach. Survey results show that STEM educators are mostly using architectural accommodations and equipment that may be already in place (e.g., ramps, LCD projector) and are less likely to be using specialized assistive technology. Although they are receiving accommodations for their primary job tasks, they are not always receiving accommodations for other aspects of their job, such as participating in professional development. Most educators are satisfied with their workplace accommodations, but almost one-third were not. In addition, many educators are determining and paying for their own accommodations, with less input from employers and rehabilitation professionals than would be expected. In order to retain educators as they age with or into disability, these issues must be addressed so that they can obtain accommodations that will effectively and comprehensively meet their workplace needs.

Background

There is a shortage of educators in subjects related to science, technology, engineering and math (STEM). School systems may address this shortage by recruiting new educators from traditionally underrepresented groups, such as people with disabilities. However, they must also find better ways to retain their existing, skilled older educators, including those who may be experiencing functional limitations due to aging.

According to the National Science Foundation, 8.8 percent of STEM educators, or 55,500, have a disability [1]. However, in a study of educators' career progression, the Scottish Council for Research in Education Centre found that educators with disabilities were more likely than other groups to think about leaving the profession (72 percent of educators with disabilities compared to 54 percent of other educators) [2]. Changes in policies, administrative attitudes, and support systems are needed to help these educators continue in their careers.

One factor that may help in the retention of educators with disabilities is the use of workplace accommodations [3, 4]. Workplace accommodations are mandated by the Americans with

Disabilities Act (ADA) as a way to provide equal opportunities for employees with disabilities [5]. They are strategies, environmental modifications or assistive technology that help a person perform a job task that he or she might otherwise not be able to perform or not perform as effectively. A national survey of employees with disabilities found that, in order to perform all of their job duties, 75 percent of the respondents needed workplace accommodations [6]. Similarly, a study of Californians with disabilities found that almost two-thirds of respondents benefited from the presence of assistive technology (AT) in the workplace [7]. Examples of accommodations for a STEM educator, including those who are aging with a disability or aging into a disability, may include the use of an interpreter at a job interview, wheelchair accessible lab furnishings, electronic spell checkers, or the provision of large print handouts during faculty meetings or seminars.

However, it is unclear what accommodations educators with disabilities are actually using and what process was followed to obtain them. Knowing this information could help other educators enter STEM education, return to work after acquiring a disability, or to counter the difficulties in performing work tasks due to aging. To investigate these questions, a national survey of K-12 and postsecondary STEM educators with a disability was conducted. This paper examines the accommodation experiences of respondents who were 55 or older and thus, were beginning to age with or into disability.

Methods and Respondent Characteristics

The online survey for educators with disabilities was advertised via a mass mailing to K-12 science and math coordinators and human resources personnel. In addition, recruitment took place through various professional organizations, including: NSTA (science teachers), AAPT (physics teachers), ITEA (technology educators), and the Educators with Disabilities Caucus. Finally, groups that are working with students with disabilities were contacted, including the Association for Higher Education and Disability, Science for Students with Disabilities, and the Educational Leadership Network of the ADA Information Centers (DBTACs). The survey took about twenty minutes to complete and included 41 questions on demographics, the subject and grades taught, barriers encountered, workplace accommodations used, and the process for receiving accommodations [8].

Table 1. Respondent functional limitations by age group

Functional Limitation	Older Educators (Age 55+)	Younger Educators (Under 55)
Physical disability	65%	68%
Hard of hearing / deaf	35%	10%
Cognitive disability	13%	36%
Health issue	13%	8%
Low vision / blind	9%	12%
Speech limitation	4%	8%

Eighty STEM educators with disabilities from 29 states or provinces completed the survey. Twenty-four of these respondents were age 55 or older. Of these, ten had become disabled prior to age 20 (and prior to becoming employed as an educator); nine had become disabled when they were 40 or older. They were established in their careers and had an average of 21 years teaching experience (standard deviation nine years). Seventy-five percent of these respondents taught science, 33 percent taught math, 13 percent taught technology or engineering, and 13 percent taught other related subjects such as medicine or economics. Forty-six percent taught grades 7-12, 33 percent taught college, 25 percent taught grades K-6, and 21 percent taught technical / community college. Respondents could list more than one option for these questions. Almost all (91 percent) taught in public, non-disability-specific schools.

Respondents were asked to report what functional limitations they were experiencing and they could list more than one limitation. As shown in Table 1, the majority (65 percent) of the older educators had a physical disability. Compared to the younger educators, a greater percent of the older respondents were hard of hearing or deaf, but fewer reported cognitive limitations such as learning disabilities or ADD. Other responses included health issues (e.g., diabetes, kidney failure) (13 percent), vision (9 percent), and speech limitations (4 percent). All but one of the older educators had told their employer that they have a disability (4 percent had not disclosed); six (12 percent) of the younger educators had not disclosed. Among those who had disclosed, slightly more than half waited to disclose until after they had started their jobs.

Results

Accommodations Used

Participants were asked what types of accommodations they used to perform their job. The most frequently used accommodations fit into the category of "universal design." They are equipment and strategies that are designed to be usable by anyone, even if a person has a functional limitation. Thus, some respondents may have reported using these products, but not specifically because they had a disability that required that accommodation. Some of these accommodations included general computer use (79 percent), use of an LCD projector or overhead projector (67 percent each) for lectures, and rearranged furniture for better accessibility (58 percent).

Other frequently reported accommodations were for architectural barriers. These included accessible parking (71 percent), hand rails (67 percent), accessible restroom (58 percent), ramps (54 percent), automatic outer doors (54 percent), and elevator (50 percent). The high use of these particular accommodations may be related to the high proportion of respondents with physical disabilities.

In contrast, most of the accommodations that are unique to STEM were infrequently reported. In fact, many of the laboratory accommodations (e.g., accessible calculators (21 percent), accessible fume hood (17 percent), and talking or tactile measurement devices (8 percent each)) were among the least frequently used.

In general, similar rates of accommodation use were found between both age groups, though several trends were noted. The older worker group, which also had a higher proportion of educators who were deaf or hard of hearing, reported a higher use of other methods for communicating (e.g., written communication), hearing aids or assistive listening devices, and amplified phones. The younger group, which had a higher proportion of educators with cognitive difficulties, reported a higher use of alternative document formats (e.g., electronic or taped documents). In addition, there was a slight trend toward lower use of accommodations for low vision among the older educators.

The younger and older educators were equally satisfied with the accommodations that they used. Among the older educators, 38 percent rated their accommodations as "good" or "excellent," 33 percent rated their accommodations as "average," and 29 percent rated their accommodations as "poor" or "very poor." It was not clear from our study whether the poorly-rated accommodations represented inappropriate accommodation selections for the needs of the individual or whether they were technologies or strategies that simply did not work.

Challenges on the Job

Respondents were presented with a list of various aspects of employment (e.g., finding job opportunities, interviewing) and were asked to indicate which ones had "negatively impacted their work experience." The results are shown in Figure 1.

Over a third of the respondents said that their disability was not a barrier to their employment. They were able to find employment, meet job requirements, and advance professionally. However, several aspects of employment were reported as challenges for many older educators, and these barriers may have been due to attitudes and/or unmet accommodation needs.

One of the most frequently reported barriers was participating in professional development (27 percent for older educators). Focus groups with K-12 educators [8] identified specific barriers that included inaccessible venues for in-service training and lack of interpreters. Accessibility of on-line and multimedia materials was also an issue, particularly for distance education.

Being promoted was the other most frequently reported barrier (27 percent). Focus group participants [8] reported that they were often reluctant to try for new job openings when they suspected that they would encounter attitudinal or architectural barriers. It was easier and safer to stay in their existing jobs. One survey respondent noted that both her dean and president were in inaccessible offices. Not being able to meet with school administrators could impact promotion opportunities.

Older educators were somewhat less likely to encounter barriers related to finding jobs and meeting job requirements, but were more likely to encounter barriers related to getting assigned to teach advanced classes. This difference between the age groups is most likely due to the older educators being more established in their careers than the younger educators.

In a separate question, educators were asked if they had ever been fired due to not having the accommodations that they needed in order to perform the job. Younger educators were more likely (14 percent) to report this problem compared to the older educators (4 percent), though this difference was not statistically significant.

Participants in the Accommodation Process

Finally, the survey included questions about who had been involved in the process of determining what accommodations would be used by the educator, and who had paid for the accommodations. The findings are shown in Table 2, excluding the three older respondents and nine younger respondents who did not use accommodations. It should also be noted that when asked how much their primary accommodation cost, the educators reported a range of "nothing" to "over $5000," with a median response of "$500-$999."

Accommodation decisions were made primarily by the educators themselves. Employers, who are supposed to have the final decision in making reasonable accommodations, were involved in the decision-making process in only 55 percent of the cases. Rehabilitation providers (e.g., vocational rehabilitation, therapists) played a limited role in the accommodation process. For 21 percent of the older educators, accommodations were solely self-determined. Overall, the findings were similar between younger and older educators.

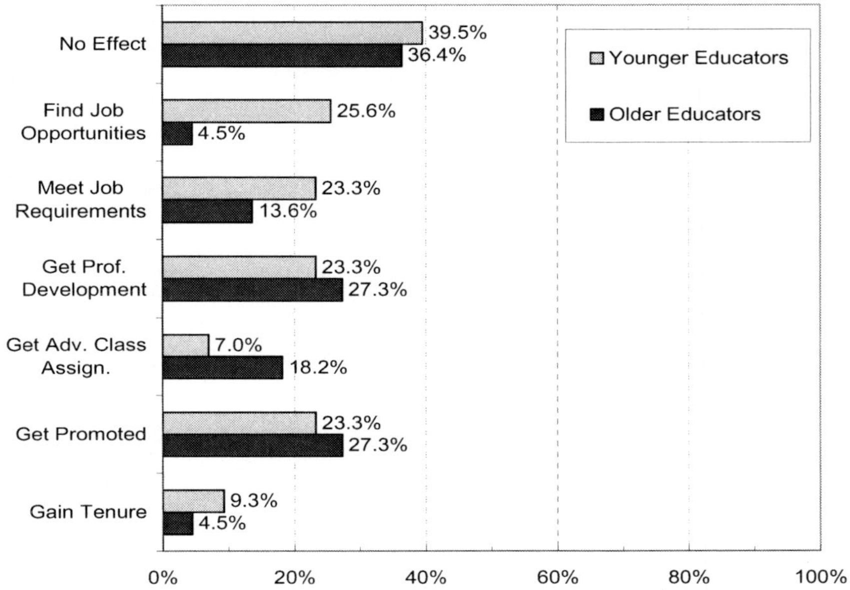

Figure 1. Employment Barriers Reported

Table 2. Involvement in Accommodation Decisions and Payment

	Involved in Decisions		Involved in Payment	
	Age 55+	**Under 55**	**Age 55+**	**Under 55**
Educator	90.9%	95.6%	65.0%	69.0%
Employer / School Administration	54.5%	53.3%	70.0%	45.2%
Medical Professional (MD, OT, PT)	13.6%	13.3%	-	-
Vocational Rehab. Services	13.6%	11.1%	15.0%	11.9%
Family / Friends / Community	9.1%	8.9%	5.0%	2.4%
Private Insurance	4.5%	4.4%	10.0%	7.1%
Co-Workers	-	6.7%	-	-
Workers Compensation Insurance	-	2.2%	5.0%	2.4%

When it came time to pay for accommodations, the educator covered at least part of the expense two-thirds of the time. Eight percent paid for all of their accommodations (compared to 27 percent of the younger educators). Employers contributed payment 70 percent of the time (compared to only 45 percent of the time for younger educators). These trends of less employer involvement and more self-reliance among younger workers did not represent statistically significant differences. Vocational rehabilitation services paid 15 percent of the time; private insurance paid 10 percent of the time.

Conclusions

According to the ADA, the process for determining accommodations should be interactive, and involve both the employee and the employer. Instead, we found that educators with disabilities often manage on their own, without accommodation support of others. For 21 percent of the older educators, accommodations were solely self-determined. Since accommodation specialists were consulted in few of the cases, the educators may not have had all of the information that they needed in order to make informed decisions about accommodations. For example, those individuals who reported that they were not satisfied with their accommodations may be trying to use strategies or technologies that are not appropriate for their needs.

Most of the accommodations that the educators reported using were those which might already be in place or which are readily available "off-the-shelf." Equipment such as a computer or LCD projector may already be commonplace within a classroom setting and not require a special request for a workplace accommodation. Accommodations related to architectural barriers may have already been put in place due to requirements of the ADA and Rehabilitation Act. In contrast, the use of specialized AT was less common, and laboratory accommodations were among the least frequently used. It was not clear from the study whether this was because the educators did not need to perform these tasks, or whether they were not aware of these accommodation options. Differences in accommodation use between age groups could be attributed primarily to differences in the functional limitations present in each sample subset.

The survey also highlighted the fact that accommodations are necessary not only for completing normal work tasks, but are also needed for other aspects of employment, such as participating in professional development and meeting with administrators. In addition, accommodation needs may be ongoing, particularly if an educator is going to have the opportunity to explore other teaching positions or class assignments.

Although the ADA places the responsibility of providing accommodations on the employer, 69 percent of the educators were paying for at least part of their accommodation needs. For comparison, a study conducted by the Work RERC across a variety of occupations found that 46 percent of the respondents paid for at least part of their accommodations [9]. We do not yet know if this increased trend toward placing payment responsibilities on the employee is unique to educators, who often are also forced to purchase their own classroom supplies.

Many educators are paying for their own accommodations because they may not wish to ask their employer for this support. The results of a recent survey conducted by the RRTC on Blindness and Low Vision on employees with disabilities found that among those respondents who needed accommodations but did not request them, 30 percent felt it was too much trouble to ask for an accommodation [10]. Thirteen percent each felt that they would not receive their requested accommodation, did not feel comfortable making a request, or were concerned about retaliation. Many of these concerns were echoed by our focus group participants. This may also be a reason why our findings showed that younger educators were less likely to have employers involved in the accommodation process and were less likely to disclose their disability to their employer. These younger educators, who are less established in their career or who in our demographics were more likely to have a learning disability, may be more reluctant to draw attention to their disability.

However, once an educator with a disability decides to request an accommodation from his or her employer, school administrators need to be made aware of their legal obligations to provide reasonable accommodations. This does not always happen. Karp and Keller's research on the career experiences of twenty-five educators with disabilities found only 56 percent who were "generally satisfied with the support, resources, adaptations, and/or accommodations used during both their preparation programs and in employment" [11]. The Scottish Council for Research in Education's study notes that "two of our disabled informants [out of 104] report that the efforts required to press for these improvements [accommodations] caused their health to deteriorate and led to them leaving teaching" [2]. Within our study, some focus group respondents reported resistance from employers to provide accommodations. In addition, although only a few educators reported having been fired due to not obtaining the accommodations that they needed, the numbers should have been zero. It is against the law to fire an employee for this reason if a reasonable accommodation exists.

In order to retain educators as they age with or into disability, these issues must be addressed so that educators can obtain workplace accommodations that will effectively and comprehensively meet their needs. It is clear that employers and educators need to understand their rights and responsibilities for accommodation. In addition, educators may not be aware of all of their accommodation options, such as specialized accommodations for laboratory tasks. To address these needs, this project is developing resources for educators and administrators on workplace accommodations.

Acknowlegements

This study was funded by grant #0435675 from the Research in Disabilities Education (RDE) program of the National Science Foundation, in partnership with the Rehabilitation Engineering Research Center on Workplace Accommodations (grant #H133E020720 / H133E070026, NIDRR, U.S. Department of Education).

References

[1] National Science Foundation (2002). Women, Minorities, and Persons with Disabilities in Science and Engineering. Arlington, VA.

[2] Powney, J., et al. (1999). Teachers' Careers: The Impact of Age, Disability, Ethnicity, Gender and Sexual Orientation, in Research Report. 2003, Scottish Council for Research in Education.

[3] Unger, D. and J. Kregel (2003). Employers' knowledge and utilization of accommodations. Work, 21(1): p. 5-15.

[4] Blanck, P.D. (1994). Communicating the Americans with Disabilities Act, Transcending Compliance: A Case Report on Sears, Roebuck and Co. Annenberg Washington Program: Iowa City. p. 69.

[5] Americans with Disabilities Act, in 42 U.S.C. § 12111 (10)(A).

[6] Williams, M., D. Sabata, and J. Zolna (2006). User needs evaluation of workplace accommodations. Work, 27(4): p. 355-362.

[7] Yeager, P., H., et al. (2006). Assistive technology and employment: Experiences of Californians with disabilities. Work, 27(4): p. 333-344.

[8] Milchus, K. (2007). Work Experience of Educators: Policy Implications for Accommodating Professionals. Proceedings of the 2007 Technology & Persons with Disability Conference, Los Angeles, CA.

[9] Milchus, K. (2007). Workplace Accommodations for Educators with Disabilities. Proceedings of the RESNA 30th Annual International Conference, Phoenix, AZ.

[10] Frank, J. J. (2006). A Survey of the Americans with Disabilities Act (ADA) Accommodation Request Experience of Persons Who are Blind or Who Have a Severe Visual Impairment. Rehabilitation Research & Training Center on Blindness & Low Vision, Mississippi State, MS.

[11] Karp, J.M. and C.E. Keller (1998). Preparation and Employment Experiences of Educators with Disabilities, in Enhancing Diversity: Educators with Disabilities, R.J. Anderson, C.E. Keller, and J.M. Karp, Editors. Gallaudet University Press: Washington, DC. p. 74-88.

Aging, Disability and Independence
W.C. Mann (Ed.)
IOS Press, 2008

doi:10.3233/978-1-58603-902-8-151

Working Posture Preferences for Elderly Computer Operators with Low Back Pain

Scott Haynes, MBME
Center for Assistive Technology and Environmental Access, Georgia Institute of Technology, Atlanta, GA USA

Abstract. Employers are looking for ways to retain older employees past retirement age. Changes in computer technology and improvements to ergonomics in the workplace make changes to traditional computer workstations more feasible. In response to these trends a study was conducted in which computer operators worked from five different postures. Results indicate that adjustments to arm supports and placement of computer peripherals impacts posture preferences, and that age-related trends warrant further research into this topic.

Keywords. Computer working postures, supine, elderly, low back pain

Introduction

There have been numerous reports citing the impact that an ageing population may have on the current workforce [2][5][11]. With the expectation that too many employees will reach the age of retirement at the same time, many employers are looking for ways to keep their employees past the typical retirement age [1][10]. As employers seek to retain their elderly employees, improvements to the work environment can play a big role.

One way in which improvements to the work environment may affect employment is in regard to people with chronic low back pain (LBP). It is estimated that 59% of people will experience LBP during their lifetime, with a peak prevalence between the ages of 45 and 59 [6]. Nearly 30% of the population will have experienced an episode of LBP by the age of 30 [4]. The configuration of typical VDT workstations not only hinders the use by some people with chronic LBP but has been shown to cause LBP after prolonged use [3].

Advances in computer technology such as lighter weight monitors, increased computing power, and advances in keyboard and mouse technology coupled with an increased awareness of workplace ergonomics allows for a greater number of options for alternative working postures for people with LBP [7]. However, very little has been written regarding computer operation from postures that differ significantly from the traditional upright posture. Some tests such as the one conducted by Monroe et al., [8] compared the use of a split keyboard and a standard (straight) keyboard in both a reclined and an upright posture as they related to typing performance and user comfort. This test was limited in its investigation of alternative working postures by the seating system, which could not move into positions such as lying fully supine or sitting with a significant backward seat pan tilt. In response to these age-related trends, and in an effort to increase employment opportunities for people with chronic low back pain, a study was conducted at the Center for Assistive Technology and Environmental Access (CATEA), in which participants performed a series of typing exercises from 5 different postures ranging from upright to lying on one's back (supine). As a part of that study, participants ranked their preferences for working posture (in the context of the study) both directly and indirectly. The purpose of this paper is to discuss the posture preferences for the participants of this study and to investigate differences between the responses of people 50 years of age or older and people under 50 years of age.

Methods

Test Design

The test was designed to be a single-factor repeated measures test in which three five-minute typing exercises would be completed in each of five different, randomly ordered working postures. The postures included Upright, Tilted, Reclined, Tilt-Recline, and Full-Recline. Table 1 describes the seating angles for each of the five different postures.

During the test, participants used two different methods to indicate their postural preferences. The first method was based on a modified Shackel Comfort scale [9]. The Shackel comfort scale

Table 1: Chair seat tilt and seat back recline angle settings (degrees).

Posture	Seat Angle [a]	Back Angle [b]	Seat to Back Angle
Upright	5	75	100
Tilted	40	40	100
Reclined	5	50	125
Tilt-Recline	40	15	125
Full-Recline	5	15	160

[a] measured from front horizontal plane
[b] measured from rear horizontal plane

allows the participants to indicate their overall comfort (OC) by selecting the appropriate point along a line marked by eleven descriptions of their level of comfort. The descriptions range from, "I feel completely relaxed," through, "I feel restless and fidgety," all the way up to, "I feel unbearable pain." A number between 0.0 and 10.0, corresponding to the location of the participant's "mark" along that line, is recorded as the OC score. The second method for indicating postural preference was based on a forced ranking from each participant of their preferences for working posture after they had completed the typing exercises in all five of the postures.

The data collection for this study occurred in two distinct phases.

- Phase 1 (Nov. '05 – April '06) was conducted by positioning the chair supports and computer components according to the participant preferences in the Upright posture. The relative position of these components remained consistent throughout all of the typing exercises for each of the 5 postures.
- Phase 2 (Feb. '07 – July '07) was conducted by re-adjusting the position of the chair supports and computer components after each typing exercise in order to maximize the comfort of the participant in each posture.

2.2 Subject recruitment

An effort was made to include a mixture of participants who had no difficulty sitting and participants who self-identified as having, "chronic recurring episodes of LBP or discomfort while sitting and working on a computer." The following inclusion criteria were used. Participants must be able to touch type, must use their computer an average of at least 10 hours per week, must be ambulatory, and must weigh less than 250 lbs. (a restriction of the test fixture used for this study). Table 2 shows the number of participants for each phase of testing grouped according to their age.

Table 2: Number of participants

Test Phase	Age < 50 yr.	Age ≥ 50 yr.
Phase 1	21	5
Phase 2	21	7
TOTAL	42	12

It is important to note that, because age-related differences were not the priority of this study, no effort was made to balance the participation of people with LBP under 50 years old and people with LBP 50 years or older. As a result, all of the participants for this study who were 50 years or older presented with issues relating to chronic LBP.

Results

To begin with, the forced ranking data from both test phases and all ages were combined into one data set. The frequency distribution for the forced ranking data is displayed in Figure 1 with error bars indicating the 95% confidence interval of ±2.6%. This figure shows that the Upright posture was the most frequently selected "favorite" posture at 37%, followed by Reclined at 31.3% and Tilted at 26.1%. The most frequently selected "least favorite" posture was Full-Recline at 44.7%, followed by Tilt-Recline at 30.4%.

A non-parametric Wilcoxon signed ranks test was conducted to compare the forced rank data with the OC data for each posture. As mentioned before, the OC score was a continuous variable with values ranging between 0.0 and 10.0. In order to compare these numbers with the forced rank data, the OC data was converted into a 1-5 ranking for each participant. Speaman's rank order correlations were calculated for the paired rankings for the five postures. All posture ranking pairs were significantly correlated except for the Full-Recline posture. No significant differences were found between the forced ranking and the ranked OC scores ($p>0.05$) when tested with a Wilcoxon statistic. Both tests demonstrate the agreement of the two measures and therefore support the validity of the forced ranking data summarized in Figure 1.

Next, the forced rank and the ranked OC scores were tested for differences between the two specified age groups. Non-parametric Mann-Whitney tests were used with no significant differences found between the specified age groups for any of the five postures, except for a weak ($p=0.049$) finding for the Upright ranked OC score.

By definition, some information related to the variability of the OC data is lost when the Spearman's rank order method is used to force the OC continuous variable into a 1-5 discrete scale. Therefore, a general linear model repeated measure analysis was

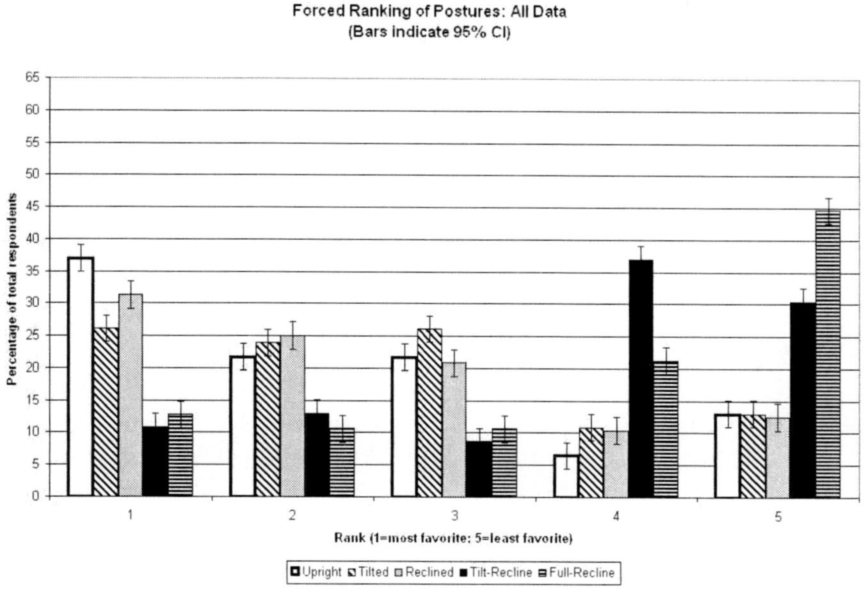

Figure 1: Summary of forced ranking of postures for all participants in both test phases.

conducted on the raw OC scores for all participants. Significant differences in the mean OC scores were indicated based on posture, $F(4,204)=2.594$ ($p<0.05$). However, there were no significant interactions indicated between posture and age at the main effect level, $F(4,204)=1.226$ ($p>0.05$). This finding supports the results of the non-parametric testing of a lack of interaction between age group and postural preference. Even though there were no significant interactions indicated, a mean plot was generated to show the mean comfort scores for each posture based on the two age groups (Figure 2). The mean plot indicated some interesting trends in the way that the older group ranked the Upright and Full-Recline postures. To further examine these trends a one-way ANOVA was run with age grouping as the independent variable. The ANOVA confirmed what is shown in the plot, that the comfort scores for Upright posture were significantly different for older participants $F(1,52)=11.258$ ($p<0.05$).

In addition to looking for differences between the two age groups, tests were run to compare results from the two phases of testing. Once again, the non-parametric Mann-Whitney tests were used and they confirmed that there was a significant difference in the way that the participants ranked the Upright postures ($p<0.05$) when the adjustments were optimized for comfort. In the first phase of testing, Upright posture was the favorite posture (mean rank=17.42) and Tilted posture was the least favorite (mean rank=27.42). In the second phase of testing Upright posture was the least favorite (mean rank=27.78) and Tilted was the favorite posture (mean rank=20.74). The percentage breakdown for the ranking of each posture for the first and second phases of testing is illustrated in Figures 3 (a) and (b) respectively.

Discussion

The summarized forced rank data demonstrated in Figure 1 indicates that in general, the Upright posture is the preferred posture and the Tilt-Recline or Full-Recline postures are the least preferred. The fact that the forced rank data correlates so closely with the ranked OC data supports the validity of the forced rank selections. However, a closer look at the data based on specified age groupings revealed a possible difference in the way that participants 50+ years old ranked the Upright posture. More of the older participants preferred the Tilted or Reclined postures to the Upright posture according to the mean plot of raw OC scores shown in Figure 2. Furthermore, there is an indication that, in general, the effort of adjusting computer peripherals and

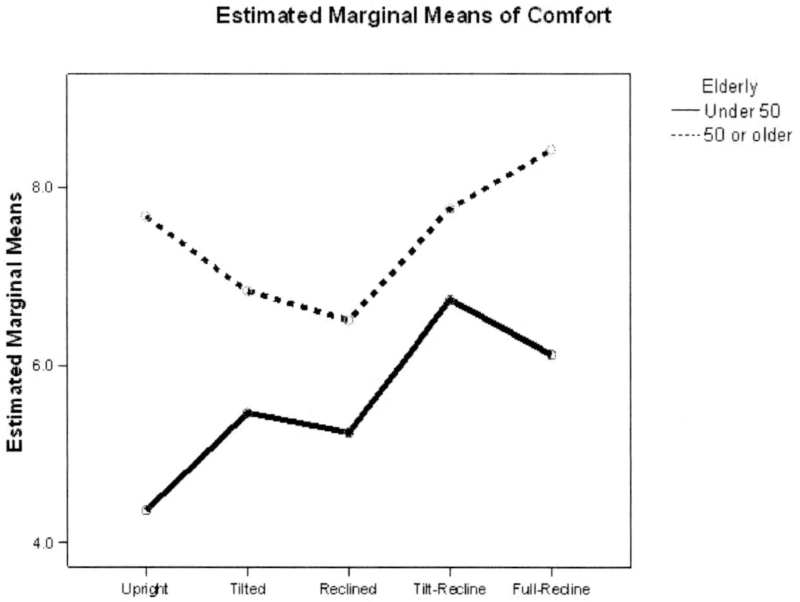

Figure 2: Estimated marginal means of raw overall comfort (OC) scores split by specified age groups.

arm supports has a significantly positive impact on the preferred ranking of alternative working postures as compared to the traditional Upright posture. Figure 3 shows that the percentage of people who selected Upright as their favorite posture dropped significantly from the Phase 1 test group to the Phase 2 test group. In general, it appears from Figure 3(a) that the Phase 1 test group

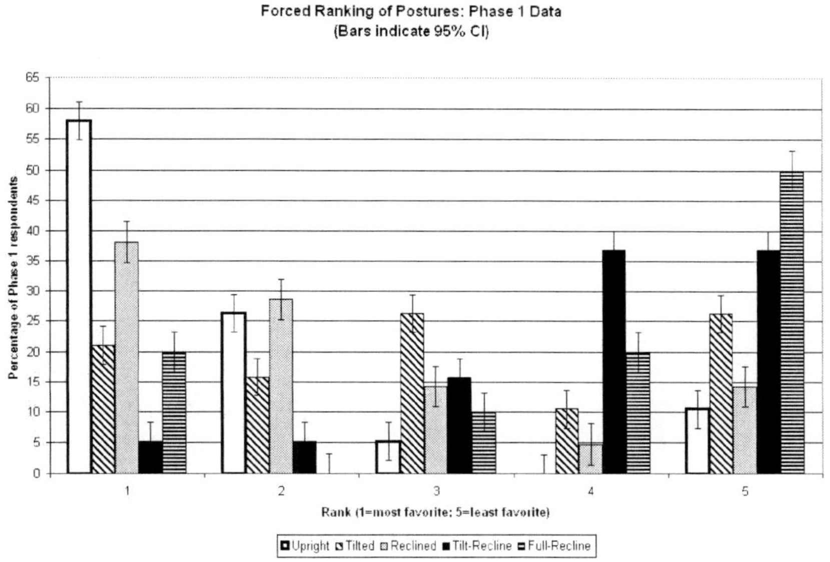

Figure 3: Frequency distribution of posture rankings for; (a) phase 1 and (b) phase 2 test groups.

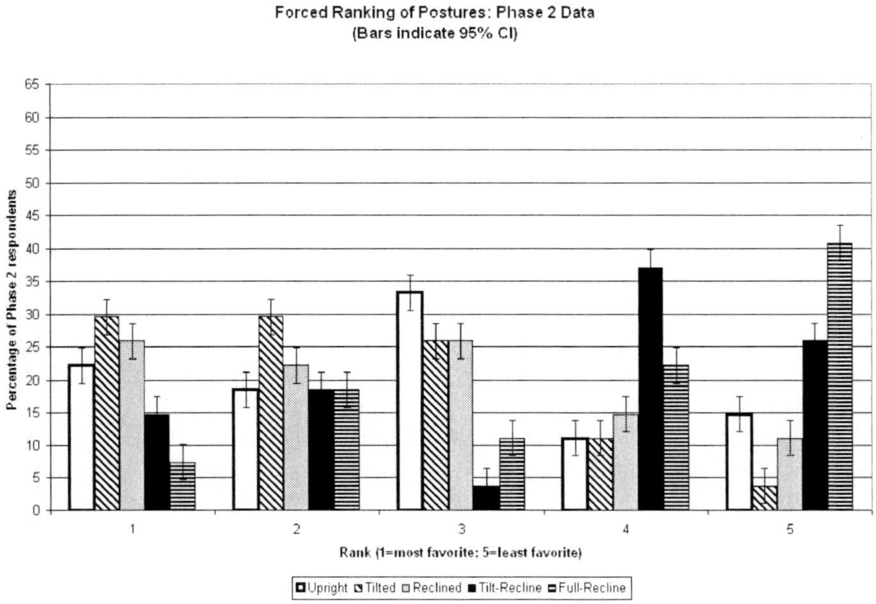

had strong opinions about the most favorite and least favorite postures. While Figure 3(b), with optimized adjustments, shows that the Phase 2 test group seemed to give higher ranking to some of the alternative postures.

One of the limitations of this study is the fact that all of the people in the older age group self-identified as having problems with LBP when sitting and working at a computer. Therefore, one may not be able to generalize these results to people 50+ years old who do not have issues with LBP. Given the nature of human subject research related to people with disabilities, it is difficult to make generalizations even about the population of people with those particular disabilities. The impact of disabling conditions on each person is so varied that a large sample size is required to make solid generalizations while taking into account all of the possible co-variants. Therefore, the relatively small sample size of participants in this study is also a limitation of this analysis.

Conclusions

The results of this data analysis so far indicate that, although Upright was the preferred working posture for participants in general, optimizing the computer peripheral placement and the arm support adjustments can significantly change the preferences for working posture. There is also an indication, based on raw OC scores, that older workers with LBP may prefer a Tilted or Reclined posture to that of a traditional Upright posture. These trends warrant further investigation into monitor and keyboard placement devices, as well as increased adjustment ranges of typical office chair seating systems for accommodating the needs of older workers with or without LBP.

Acknowledgements

The author would like to acknowledge Bill Del'Aune for his help in regard to the statistical data analysis. This research was supported through the Rehabilitation Engineering Research Center (RERC) on Workplace Accommodations, which is supported by Grant H133E020720 of the National Institute on Disability and Rehabilitation Research of the U.S. Department of Education. The opinions contained in this paper are those of the grantee and do not necessarily reflect those of the U.S. Department of Education.

References

[1] Armstrong-Stassen, M., & Templer, A. J. (2006). The Response of Canadian Public and Private Sector Human Resource Professionals to the Challenge of the Aging Workforce. Public Personnel Management, 35(3), 247.

[2] Arnone, W. J. (2006). Are Employers Prepared for the Aging of the U.S. Workforce? Benefits Quarterly, 22(4), 7.

[3] Bendix, T. (1994). Low back pain and seating. In R. Lueder & K. Noro (Eds.), Hard Facts about Soft Machines - The Ergonomics of Seating (pp. 147-155). London: Taylor & Francis Ltd.

[4] Croft, P. R., Macfarlane, G. J., Papageorgiou, A. C., Thomas, E., & Silman, A. J. (1998). Outcome of low back pain in general practice: a prospective study. British medical journal, 316(7141), 1356-1359.

[5] Eisen, P. (2003). Keeping America Competitive -- How a Talent Shortage Threatens U.S. Manufacturing (White Paper). Washington, D.C.: National Association of Manufacturers, The Manufacturing Institute, and Deloitte & Touche.

[6] Frank, A. O. (2002). Back pain. Rheumatology (Oxford), 41(9), 1069-1070.

[7] Haynes, S., & Williams, K. (2007). Product Review of Alternative Computer Workstations as Possible Workplace Accommodations for People with Chronic Low Back Pain. Technology and Disability, 19(1), 41-52.

[8] Monroe, M. J., Sommerich, C. M., & Mirka, G. A. (2001). The influence of head, forearm and back support on myoelectric activity, performance and subjective comfort during a VDT task. Paper presented at the Human Factors and Ergonomics Society 45th Annual Meeting, Minneapolis/ St.Paul, MN, United States.

[9] Shackel, B., Chidsey, K. D., & Shipley, P. (1969). The Assessment of Chair Comfort. Ergonomics, 12(2), 269-306.

[10] Waters, T. R., & MacDonald, L. A. (2001). Ergonomic job design to accommodate and prevent musculoskeletal disabilities. Assistive Technology, 13(2), 88-93.

[11] Wolozin, H. (1985). Corporate Power in an Aging Economy: Labor Force Policy Corporate Power in an Aging Economy: Labor Force Policy. Journal of Economic Issues, 19(2), 475.

Aging, Disability and Independence
W.C. Mann (Ed.)
IOS Press, 2008

doi:10.3233/978-1-58603-902-8-161

Policy Change and the Accommodating Workplace: Issues, Barriers, and Opportunities

Paul M.A. Baker, Ph.D., AICP[1], Nathan W. Moon, M.S.[1]
[1]Workplace Accommodations RERC /Center for Advanced Communications Policy (CACP), Georgia Institute of Technology, Atlanta, GA 30332, USA

Abstract: A conceptual framework of workplace accommodation issues associated with the employment of people with disabilities and the aging was developed to help identify policy barriers and opportunities, using online policy Delphi Method, an iterative polling instrument used to assess key issues and intervention options. This paper presents the results of research conducted toward articulating policy initiatives that address the key issues critical to the development of effective approaches for the implementation of workplace accommodations.

Introduction

A number of significant social, economic, technological, and policy barriers exist to full integration of people with disabilities into the work environment and opportunities for their employment. According to the U.S. Department of Labor (DOL), "Americans with disabilities are active and contributing members of our society and they must have the opportunity to develop the skills they need to compete and obtain jobs in the 21st century workforce" [19]. Information from the 1996 Panel of the Survey of Income and Program Participation (SIPP) found that 7.2 million individuals with a disability between the ages of 15-64 were able to work but experienced limitations in the type of work they could do [3]. According to the U.S. Census, there is a 14.1 percent unemployment rate among persons with disabilities, as compared to an unemployment rate of 5.8 percent for people without disabilities [27]. Policymakers have attempted to reduce barriers to employment for people with disabilities; however, the persistent population of unemployed and under-employed people with disabilities, and the increasingly aging workforce, remains a problem. The innovation and implementation of appropriate workplace accommodations is one approach that has been used to reach the goal of equal employment opportunity for people with disabilities. Successful workplace accommodations can incorporate an array of solutions ranging from: new assistive devices, and universally-designed technologies to employment activity and process approaches, and policy initiatives at the employer and governmental levels.

A conceptual framework of workplace accommodation issues associated with the employment of people with disabilities and the aging was developed to help identify policy barriers and opportunities, using online policy Delphi Method, a polling instrument used to assess key issues and intervention options. This paper presents the results of research conducted toward articulating policy initiatives that address the key issues critical to the development of effective approaches for the implementation of workplace accommodations.

Conceptual Framework

A key finding from the Workplace Accommodations RERC is that, as a policy research area, the objective of ensuring that appropriate workplace accommodations are made poses several interesting problems. Policies that support the development of workplaces that can accommodate all characteristics and abilities of individuals cross a wide variety of legal, policy, technological, social, and human factors issues. From the perspective of social scientists, as well as policy makers, the failure to integrate people with disabilities into the workplace has two implications. First, at the level of the disabled person, the failure often leads to diminished degree of social contacts and social support (social capital). This, in turn, can result in compromises to the health of the disabled person beyond purely disability related ones. Second, at the level of the community (or society) this failure often leads to a widening in the gap between those with access to social capital and those without (or having less) access to social capital. The widening of this gap can lead to a larger, systemic breakdown of social cohesion, and a general lowering of the level of health present in the community (society). Therefore it is important to identify people with disabilities, as well as create public (employment and health) policies that promote their integration into the workplace (and so too, into the larger communities in which the various workplaces exist).

To this end, this project explored approaches to the use of policy as a cross-disciplinary vehicle for achieving improved workplace conditions. A conceptual framework (see Table 1) of accommodations that can be adapted to the workplace is structured around an identification of "themes" or crosscutting components (e.g. data collection, accommodation practices, the aging worker, emergency communications, etc.). These are then further broken down into associated barriers (access, economic, policy/regulatory, environmental, awareness, social, technological) and their impact on workplace, stakeholders, policy-related approaches to addressing the problems, and potential outcomes from problem resolution. The matrix serves as an organizing heuristic to help focus policy related approaches to problem solution.

Initial results from the Workplace Accommodation RERC's Policy Delphi further probes five important issues related to workplace accommodations: 1) Emergency preparedness and safety in the workplace for persons with disabilities; 2) Inadequate/insufficient data on the incidence, nature, and cost of workplace accommodations; 3) Incomplete employer understanding/awareness of workplace accommodations; 4) Telework as an accommodation for persons with disabilities; and 5) Aging as an issue of increasing salience regarding the U.S. workforce and the importance of addressing the needs of aging persons with disability and workers aging into disability. These topics are elaborated upon below, and represent key thematic areas to be further investigated in the ongoing RERC research.

Key Barriers/Issues

A literature review of workplace accommodations [3]revealed some key types of barriers that are common to most policy issues (including the ones previously identified). These include: awareness/access, economic, environmental, and regulatory/policy, social and technological barriers, which manifest in an employment context as issues that impact the employee, employer, workplace setting, or the general understanding of the nature of accommodations or disability, per se. A more detailed discussion of these follows.

Data Collection on Employment of PWD, Workplace Accommodation & Integration

A major problem with developing policy to address disability related issues in general, as well as the specific issues of workplace accommodations, is the insufficiency of available data capturing the nature and circumstances of workplace accommodations [8]

[9] [17] [18] [24] . Further, the data that is available may be misrepresenting the current state of employment and workplace accommodations implementation among individuals with disabilities. The survey methodologies that are used currently to account for people with disabilities who are employed may be slightly skewed, as they may not accurately account for all workers who have disabilities. The data on the implementation of workplace accommodations within the United States also fails to fully incorporate the views of employers, especially those who have never employed an individual with a disability [25].

Range of Accommodations

As noted above, workplace accommodations involve changes to the work environment that are typically practice-related, technological, or environmental in nature. Universal design and assistive technologies are areas of major interest within this issue sphere [12]. Frequently, employees with disabilities and their employers (or potential) lack information of available assistive technology options, applicability of process approaches such as teleworking, or even awareness that a range of accommodations exist. Further, there is a concern that due to lack of awareness, manufacturers of workplace related devices or technologies (i.e. information and communication devices, software, telephones, etc.) may not design for all users, or do not optimally design technology to be adaptable for a wider array of user characteristics. Universally designed devices would provide great benefits for workers with disabilities because they would have easier integration into the environment with less need for changes to be implemented by employers. This universal design concern can be more broadly applied to telecommunications technologies which pose barriers for some persons with disabilities and may impact their workplace options.

Of specific interest was the attention to teleworking. While telecommuting has emerged as a viable workplace accommodation for persons with disabilities [1]; telework, a distinct concept arranged entirely around a virtual workplace [4] [5], provides a means to provide such individuals with a new way for entering the workforce. The Policy Delphi strongly suggests that employers are concerned that workers will not be as productive outside the office while teleworking, a belief that is not specifically supported in extant studies. Even as the structural barriers to successful telework options have been identified, there is a need to examine in greater detail the role of employers in promoting or hindering telework as an accommodation.

Safety/Emergency Preparedness

The recent occurrence of natural disasters and other emergency situations experienced by the United States has highlighted the importance of emergency communications and preparedness planning especially for people with disabilities, and other vulnerable populations. People with disabilities face compounded vulnerabilities in the face of disaster and emergencies, due to a variety of functional and sensory limitations they may experience which makes the ability to communicate instructions and information even more critical to them.

As part of the effort to ensure that the needs of people with disabilities are integrated in emergency preparedness plans, accommodations for the workplace have become a major priority. Research over the last decade has shown that people with disabilities are often overlooked during workplace planning efforts due to lack of awareness about the needs or their responsibilities. This unawareness may also translate to fear on the part of the employer about employing those with disabilities because of liability concerns during an emergency [28].

Aging Workers

The issues of aging workers are extremely relevant to the workplace environment, particularly as the demographics of the U.S. population changes. Although aging workers experience similar barriers as people with disabilities when it comes to the workplace, their specific concerns may be slightly different. Additionally, accommodations for workers who are aging into disability are important because of the projections about the changing demographics of the work-eligible population. Issues with accommodating this group come from social barriers about the employability of aging adults. There are also issues with the existing legislative framework and the work benefits that those beyond retirement can receive [15].

Policy Options

In response to the above noted workplace issues and accommodations barriers, the literature suggests that informed implementation of policy approaches can help facilitate the development of the accommodation workplaces. Within the broad category of external (policy) interventions there are awareness, market/economic, or policy-based approaches; the specific designs chosen rely on a generalizable knowledge base. The Workplace Accommodations RERC is conducting ongoing stakeholder related research on the feasibility of currently existing policy based approaches to improving workplace accommodations, and is exploring additional options for policy development in light of stakeholder input. Initial findings suggest options which include:

- Comprehensive efforts to catalogue existing accommodations in order to provide best practice examples of existing successful workplace accommodations.
- Increased outreach efforts to encourage corporations' awareness about information resources like the Job Accommodation Network (JAN) and the World Wide Web Consortium (W3C) that provide simple steps that can be taken to accommodate people with disabilities.
- Revised federal regulations for workplace safety to incorporate changes to cover nontraditional workplace environments made possible by information technologies.
- Identification of key gaps in available training and barriers to the implementation of appropriate communication procedures will allow development of specific training modules which would be disseminated for use in emergency communications plans used by state and local and core county points of contact and coordinated with the stakeholders.
- Identification of contextual factors affecting telework as a workplace accommodation, including misunderstandings by employers of the range of telework options as an accommodation.
- Development of enhanced models of accommodation that recognize that accommodating the ageing worker is a multidimensional process that requires parsing the difference between the changing needs of younger workers with disabilities as they age, as well as those workers aging into disability and their need for accommodations.

Acknowledgements

This is a publication of the RERC on Workplace Accommodations, which is supported by Grant H133E020720 of the National Institute on Disability and Rehabilitation Research of the U.S. Department of Education. The opinions contained in this publication are those of the grantee and do not necessarily reflect those of the U.S. Department of Education.

References

[1] Anderson, J., Bricout, J. C., & West, M.D. (2001). Telecommuting: Meeting the needs of businesses and employees with disabilities. Journal of Vocational Rehabilitation, 16(2), 97-104.

[2] Baker, P. M. A. (2005). Virtual exclusion and telework: The double-edged sword of technocentric workplace accommodation policy. Paper presented at the Workplace RERC State of the Science Conference, Atlanta, Georgia.

[3] Baker, P. M. A., & Ward, A. C. (2004). Toward development of the accommodating workplace: Key technological and policy issues. Paper presented at the California State University, Northridge (CSUN) Center on Disabilities' 19th Annual International Technology and Persons with Disabilities Conference, Los Angeles, California.

[4] Baker, P. M. A., & Ward, A.C. (2006a). Telework and people with disabilities: Developing the "e-clusive" workplace. In A. Anttiroiko & M. Malkia (Eds.), Encyclopedia of Digital Government. Hershey, PA: Idea Group Publishing.

[5] Baker, P. M. A., & Ward, A. C. (2006b). Toward development of the accommodating workplace: Key technological and policy issues. Paper presented at California State University, Northridge (CSUN) Center on Disabilities' 21st Annual International Technology and Persons with Disabilities Conference, Los Angeles, California.

[6] Baker, P. M. A., Moon, N. W., & Bakowski, A. (2006). Increasing access to wireless technologies: Results of a policy Delphi study. Paper presented at California State University, Northridge (CSUN) Center on Disabilities' 21st Annual International Technology and Persons with Disabilities Conference, Los Angeles, California.

[7] Baker, P. M. A., Moon, N. W., & Ward, A. C. (2006). Virtual exclusion and telework: Barriers and opportunities of technocentric workplace accommodation policy. WORK: A Journal of Prevention, Assessment & Rehabilitation, 24(7), 421-430.

[8] Blanck, P. D. (1997). The economics of the employment provisions of the ADA: Part I: Workplace accommodations. DePaul Law Review, 46(4), 877-914.

[9] Blanck, P. D., Schur, L., Kruse, D., Schwochau, S., & Song, C. (2003). Calibrating the impact of the ADA's employment provisions. Stanford Law and Policy Review, 14(2), 267-290.

[10] Bricout, J. C. (2004). Using telework to enhance return to work outcomes for people with spinal cord injuries. NeuroRehabilitation, 19(2), 147-159.

[11] Brostrand, H. L. (2006). Tilting at windmills: Changing attitudes toward people with disabilities," Journal of Rehabilitation, 72(1), 4-9.

[12] Bruyere, S., & Erickson, W. (2005). IT and the workplace: Implications for persons with disabilities. Ithaca, N.Y.: Employment & Disability Institute, Cornell University.

[13] Dziak, M. (2005). Remote possibilities for workplace access. Paper presented at the Workplace RERC State of the Science Conference, Atlanta, Georgia.

[14] Endicott, S. (2005). Workplace accommodation outcomes. Paper presented at Workplace RERC State of the Science Conference, Atlanta, Georgia.

[15] Finch, J., & Robinson, M. (2003). Aging and late onset disability: Addressing workplace accommodation. Journal of Rehabilitation, 69(2), 38-42.

[16] Head, L. (2005). Ageing and the accommodating workplace: A survey of employer practice. Paper presented at Workplace RERC State of the Science Conference, Atlanta, Georgia.

[17] Head, L., Baker P. M. A., Bagwell, B., & Moon N. W. (2006). Barriers to evidence based practice in accommodations for an aging workforce. WORK: A Journal of Prevention, Assessment & Rehabilitation, 24(7), 391-396.

[18] Hendricks, D. J., Batiste, L. C., Hirsh, A., Schartz, H., & Blanck, P. (2005). Cost and effectiveness of accommodations in the workplace: Preliminary results of a nationwide survey. Disability Studies Quarterly, 25(4). Available at [http://www.dsq-sds.org].

[19] Job Accommodation Network. (2006). Employer's practical guide to reasonable accommodation under the Americans with Disabilities Act (ADA). Available online at [http://www.jan.wvu.edu/Erguide/One.htm#D].

[20] Kaplan, S. (2005). Telecommuting as a reasonable accommodation: A framework for decision-making. Paper presented at the Workplace RERC State of the Science Conference, Atlanta, Georgia.

[21] Mackert, R. (2002). Report on special needs – Issues, efforts and lessons learned. New York: Federal Emergency Management Agency – State Disaster Field Office. Available online at [http://www.eadassociates.com/SNreport-dr1391.doc].

[22] Robertson, M. M., Maynard, W., & McDevitt, J. (2003). Telecommuting: Managing the safety of workers in the home environment. Professional Safety, 48(4), 30-36.

[23] Sanford, J., & Milchus, K. (2006). Evidence-based practice in workplace accommodations. WORK: A Journal of Prevention, Assessment & Rehabilitation, 27(4), 329-332.

[24] Schartz, H. A., Hendricks, D. J., & Blanck, P. (2006). Workplace accommodations: Evidence based outcomes. Work: A Journal of Prevention, Assessment & Rehabilitation, 27(4), 345-354.

[25] Silverstein, R., Julnes, G., & Nolan, R. (2005). What Policymakers Need and Must Demand From Research Regarding the Employment Rate of Persons with Disabilities. Behavioral Sciences and the Law, 23(3), 399-448.

[26] Strobel, W., & McDonough, J. T. (2003). Workplace personal assistance service and assistive technology. Journal of Vocational Rehabilitation, 18(2), 107-112.

[27] U.S. Census Bureau. (2006). P70-107: Americans with disabilities: 2002. Washington, D.C. : Department of Commerce.

[28] U.S. Department of Homeland Security. (2005). Individuals with disabilities in emergency preparedness: Annual report. Washington, D.C.: Government Printing Office. Available online at [http://www.dhs.gov/xlibrary/assets/CRCL_IWDEP_AnnualReport_2005.pdf].

[29] Ward, A. C., & Baker, P. M. A. (2005). Disabilities and impairments: Strategies for workplace integration. Behavioral Sciences & the Law, 23(1), 143-160.

[30] White House Conference on Aging (WHCOA) Policy Committee. (2005). WHCOA report to the President and Congress: The booming dynamics of aging: From awareness to action. Washington, D.C.: Department of Health and Human Services. Available online at [http://www.whcoa.gov/about/about.asp#report].

Table 1: Workplace Accommodations Conceptual Policy Matrix

THEME	BARRIER TYPE	ISSUES	STAKEHOLDERS	APPROACHES	OUTCOMES
Data Collection on Employment of PWD, Workplace Accommodation & Integration (D)	Access	• Lack of data on the positive impacts of accommodating PWDs in the workplace (e.g. AT, telework (Dziak, 2005), etc.) • Scarcity of best practice examples on existing accommodations and policies • Paucity of research on WA issues from the employer perspective • Insufficient documentation on the number of jobs that employ accommodations for their employees • Specific accommodation solutions & outcomes not well documented in the literature (Endicott, 2005) • Deficiency of empirical evidence on whether older workers are being accommodated (Head, 2005) • Only a few studies that examine the effect that aging with a disability may have on employment options • Much of the literature around PWDs and employment focuses on issues & strategies for potential employees in applying for and finding work. There is much less of an emphasis on the issues for PWD who are already employed	• People with disabilities (PWD) • Researchers • Employers • Disability advocates • Government/ Public Institutions (Research)	*Document & Develop* • Provide best practice examples of existing successful WAs *Research-oriented* • Perform more surveys and case study evaluations of workplace accommodations (esp. from employer perspective) • Perform more research on employment outcomes *Economic/Market-based* • Provide incentive to employers/corporations to participate in research	• Better understanding of the current scene of workplace accommodations • Provide examples & models for other companies to follow • Greater participation from employers • Better understanding of barriers to increased employment of PWDs from the employer point of view
	Policy/Regulatory	• Discrepancies in how disability is defined and who is included for research/policy purposes • Misclassification or undercounting of the number of employed PWD by current surveys methods	• PWD • Policymakers • Researchers • Disability advocates • Government agencies	*Governmental Effort* • Assessment of existing survey tools • Development of new tools for data collection	• Improve the accuracy of existing data sets regarding PWDs & workplace accommodations which will allow for greater understanding of the current state of workplace accommodations and steps to take for the future
	Environmental	• Formal vs. informal accommodations -what defines an accommodation? There may be accommodations that are being implemented and not documented, thereby impacting the data	• PWD • Policymakers • Researchers • Government/ public institutions • Disability	*Research-oriented* • Develop a means of getting stakeholder (employers) input on the process • Modify survey methodologies to inquire about possible things that were done that	• Improve the data sets for WA regarding the types of accommodations that are being implemented • Provides a more accurate view of the

			advocates	may not have been documented	how employers are accommodating people with disabilities
Workplace Accommodations [in general] (incl. UD overall) (W)	Awareness/Access	• Employees/employers may not know what accommodating options are available • Lack of understanding of the various types of accommodations for the various disabilities • Lack of clearly defined job tasks and responsibilities (Strobel & McDonough, 2003) can impact the ability to properly assess what accommodation would be best	• Employers • PWD • Aging/Older populations • Disability advocates	• Educate PWD about their options and rights (use JAN, ODEP, etc. • Educate employers about their obligations and resources	• Reduces the misconception that PWD are a hassle or lack workable skills in the workplace • This may lead to increased employment of people with disabilities • Increases awareness about the best options for accommodation
	Social	• Misconceptions and negative perceptions of the abilities of PWDs by employers & employees (Brostrand, 2006)	• PWD • Employers • Disability advocates • Policymakers • Vocational/ Rehab specialist	*Policy-oriented*: • Develop employer relationships with voc. rehab programs such that disability/sensitivity training is involved in the outreach process • Companies can develop polices regarding the hiring of people with disabilities	• Initiate a change in attitudes of employers and co-workers through education & relationship building • Disability awareness training could become more widely used
	Technology (AT, EIT issues)	• Limitations with the scope of definitions of EIT as they apply to WA & PWDS (Baker & Ward, 2006b); Section 255 of the Federal Communications Act defines "telecommunication services" as services that facilitate and carry voice communication. This definition appears to leave e-mail and data transmission uncovered. • Concerns regarding who is responsible under the ADA for ensuring that websites & EIT are accessible for employees and/or applicants with disabilities	• PWD • Employers • EIT manufacturers • Government agencies • Vocational/ Rehab Agencies	*Policy-oriented*: • Clearly define who is responsible for things like job posting websites under the ADA • Stronger requirements for accessibility of EIT devices	• Better integration of PWD into the workplace as they can use the same equipment • Reduce digital divide for PWD which can lead to greater employment options due to access to more job postings, and information • empower a prospective AT user to have an intelligent conversation about what technology might be beneficial and what device would be the most effective for the job tasks
	Economic	• Lack of incentive for private industry to think in terms of UD for products	• Employers • PWD • Disability advocates • Manufacturers • Designers		
	Regulatory	• Devices and services not covered under private and employer-based health insurance, along with Medicare &		*Regulatory* • Government funded incentives for	

		Medicaid (Baker, Moon, & Bakowski, 2006)		companies/manufacturers to develop UD/EIT devices • Reduce income caps mandated by the federal government that may create barriers	
Safety/Emergency Preparedness (S)	Access/Awareness	• Lack of emergency egress plans that can broadly fit all employees • Emergency workers need more training on the special needs of PWD • Perception by employers that PWD are more likely to be a safety liability, in turn negatively affecting their ability to get hired. • PWDs may experience "changes" to their job status from employers who want to avoid accommodating safety/EP concerns.	• PWDs • Emergency Officials • Employers • Emergency workers • Public safety entities	• Outreach – Include PWD in the process for developing emergency plans • Educate – Train emergency officials and workers on the special needs of PWD and how to aid them in the event of an emergency (Mackert, 2002)	
	Technological	• Lack of equipment that can be used by PWD in an emergency or failure of communication systems • Technology and workspaces designed to notify PWD of emergencies should be accessible (AT or UD)	• PWDs • Manufacturers of emergency devices • Manufacturers of AT devices for emergency equipment • Employers • Public safety entities	• Provide incentives to equipment developers to use more UD approaches	
	Policy/Regulatory	• Lack of clearly defined policy that requires universal application (or as close to as possible) in emergency planning • Concerns with workplace safety of PWD who telework (Robertson, Maynard, & McDevitt, 2003) • Lack of specificity in legislation regarding telework and what responsibilities employers have •	• PWD • Aging/older populations • Policymakers • Employers • Public safety entities	*Policy-oriented* • Redefine OSHA regulations to include non-traditional work settings (such as homes)	
Aging Workers (A)	Policy/Regulatory	• Lack of incentives for employers to provide an work environment that continues to accommodate workers as they age (WHCOA, 2005) • Employers need to alter their employment terms and policies to accommodate the aging workforce • Existing legislation regarding pensions and such may discourage employers/employees from extending work beyond retirement eligibility	• Aging/Older populations • Policymakers • Employers	• Development of federal programs to encourage accommodating aging workers • Write/change existing legislations regarding retirement benefits and eligibility	• Reduces the impact the labor shortfall will have on the US economy • Educates employers about the importance of older workers to the future of work environment • Removes legislative barriers that discourage work past retirement
	Awareness	• Employers not recognizing the	• Aging/Older	• Employers need to develop	• Gives aging workers

		magnitude of the change and see no reason to make adjustments at the moment • Changing workforce demographics lead to greater percentage of older workers • Many in the aging group want to continue work into their late 50s to early 60s	populations • Policymakers • Employers • Research agencies	more flexible workplace options such as flexible hours, part time schedule, etc.	more incentive to stay in the workforce
	Economic	• Issues with large number of aging adults being supported by government benefit programs; (Finch & Robinson, 2003)	• Aging/older populations • Employers • Policymakers • Government agencies		• Reduces the number of unemployed aging individuals • Reduces the large draw on federal benefits like social security, Medicaid, etc.
	Technological	• Resistance to using technology(incl. AT) by those with late onset disability due to unfamiliarity with the technology or not accepting themselves as disabled • Lack of training resources for aging workers to learn to use technologies	• Aging/older populations • Employers • Policymakers • ICT manufacturers		
	Social	• Employers may hold negative attitudes towards keeping older workers & their abilities (corporate culture) • Older workers are less likely to find new employment if they are fired • Lack of recognition of by older individuals of themselves as "with disabilities"	• Aging/older populations • Employers • Policymakers • Government	• Educate more older people on their options and resources as they age into disability • Incorporate VR with resources for aging workers • Awareness and outreach campaigns for employers	
Telework/Telecommuting (T)	Access/Awareness	• Lack of availability of this type of accommodation; lack of knowledge about this type of accommodation by PWDs (Anderson, 2001) • Misconception on the part of the employer about actual costs of telework • Misinformation on the benefits of this kind of accommodation • Misconceptions about the effect of telework on the work environment	• Aging/Older populations • PWD • Employers	• Develop materials for knowledge dissemination to employers & employees with disabilities regarding telework • Provide cases of best practices in telecommuting • Educate policy officials about telework issues specific to PWDs	• Increase the employment numbers of PWD
	Economic	• Therefore there is an imbalance in the physical costs vs. possible benefits • Concern by employers over the costs of implementing telework(technology & other costs) • Concern that telework implementation is more expensive with PWDs (AT & such)	• PWD • Employers • Government officials • Disability advocates	• Develop/support community broadband/telecom initiatives	• Changes an employer's perception of telework and PWD • Provides a better CBA analysis of telework
	Policy/Regulatory	• Lack of consistent policies and procedures on how to evaluate what is a reasonable/flexible request for telework (Kaplan, 2005)	• PWD • Employers • Policymakers	• Develop examples & training modules to help employers foster virtual social networks • Establishment of a program to assist PWDs in obtaining	• Increased access/availability of government resources

		• Concerns about OSHA regulations & their application to this evolving work option • Lack of policy to integrate PWD into the workplace (loss of social capital) (Baker, 2005)		telework positions • Development of policies to specifically address telework for PWDs	
	Technological	• Availability of technologies that enable employees with disabilities to telework	• PWD • Employers • AT manufacturers		
	Social	• Concerns about the remote aspect of telework: lack of work support, job structure, social interaction (Baker, Moon, & Ward, 2006) • Issues with telework promoting white collar work among some PWD and "pink" collar in those with less skills	• PWD • Aging/Older populations • Disability advocates • Community leaders		
Service Delivery (SD)	Economic	• Concerns about the cost of implementing accommodations & who will do the implementing	• PWD • Employers • Disability advocates • Funding agencies Policymakers	• Outreach to employers by disability employment advocate agencies with resources such as JAN, ODEP, USBLN	• Employers feel more informed about the employment about PWDs and resources at their disposal for such a process
	Awareness/Access	• Perception by employers that it is costly in time and money to implement accommodations for PWDs	• PWD • Employers • Disability advocates • Funding agencies • Policymakers • Vocational Rehab specialist		
	Technological	• There are a number of different systems & accommodation types for all the different functional limitations. • Concerns about technological accommodation devices and the need to make sure they are compatible, maintained and upgraded (i.e., who covers this cost? Who is responsible for doing it? These are all concerns from the employer perspective.)	• PWD • Employers • Device manufacturers • Policymakers/ legislators • Funding entities /agencies • Disability advocates		

Aging, Disability and Independence
W.C. Mann (Ed.)
IOS Press, 2008

doi:10.3233/978-1-58603-902-8-175

Competitive Enablement: A Consumer-Oriented Approach to Device Selection in Device-assisted Vision Rehabilitation

Graham Strong*†; Jeffrey Jutai‡, Ann Plotkin*, Pauline Bevers*
*Centre for Sight Enhancement and School of Optometry, University of Waterloo, Waterloo, Ontario, Canada
‡Aging, Rehabilitation and Geriatric Care Research Centre, Lawson Health Research Institute, London, Ontario, Canada
† Correspondence to: J. Graham Strong, OD, MSc, Centre for Sight Enhancement, University of Waterloo, Waterloo, Ontario, Canada

Abstract: The role of device-assisted vision rehabilitation is to recommend assistive technology to ameliorate vision disabilities that people with impaired vision identify as being problematic. "Competitive enablement" is a conceptual approach wherein individual consumers evaluate the functional utility of competing device interventions while performing a series of self-identified problematic tasks of high functional relevance to the individuals themselves. Adherence to this approach lessens abandonment rates and produces significant impacts in both functional and psychosocial domains.

Background

Low vision describes any condition of diminished vision that cannot be corrected by standard eyeglasses, contact lenses, or surgical intervention, and that interferes with a person's ability to perform common, age-appropriate, seeing tasks[1]. Massof [2] notes that "a person is disabled when, because of disease, disorder, or injury, he/she has abnormal difficulty with (or cannot perform) routine activities that he/she would normally be able to do." The magnitude of the disability is simply the difference between normal ability and the current ability of the individual. This coincides with what Agree [3] describes as the "underlying disability." She defines "residual disability" as "the degree of disablement that remains after personal care or assistive devices have ameliorated some part of the total underlying need." The concept of device-mediated "enablement" then describes the difference between the underlying disability and the residual disability when using an assistive device. The role of device-assisted vision rehabilitation is to use assistive technology (AT) to improve functional performance levels so that the person can accomplish tasks of importance that are otherwise problematic. Ameliorating vision disabilities in this way helps the person maximize functional independence, improves quality of life, and facilitates adaptation to the psychosocial aspects of vision loss.4

Competitive Enablement

Competitive Enablement (CE) is a conceptual approach wherein individual consumers evaluate the functional utility of competing device interventions while performing a series of self-identified problematic tasks of high functional relevance to the individuals themselves. The concept evolves from the credible premise that no two devices provide individual users with identical levels of satisfaction, nor do any two consumers have precisely the same needs and expectations for devices they are purchasing. The proliferation of assistive device technology is making it increasingly difficult for service consumers to make effective choices within the ever-expanding range of options [5]. While there are many generic similarities between different products, there are also identifiable differences. Once it becomes apparent that an individual may benefit from using a specific type of access device, the next problem is to determine which specific product should be purchased to address this need. A CE approach requires consumers to make critical evaluations about the functional effectiveness of competing devices, while performing a series of highly relevant problematic tasks. Many different devices have the capacity to provide acceptable levels of functional performance for specific seeing tasks such as reading the newspaper. However, these devices often can be differentiated by considering other factors such as cost, ease of use, versatility, safety, universality, cosmetics, comfort, availability, serviceability, innovation, practicality, and adaptability. The significance of these various attributes will vary for different consumers. Taken alongside the performance attributes of the different devices, these considerations make it possible to identify the best device for each individual consumer. The function of the assessment process is no longer to identify a device that works for the consumer, but rather to identify the one device that works best.

Recalling the subjective decisions required in a standard eye examination provides a useful illustration of the proposed protocol. Most people are familiar with the procession of subjective comparisons that are offered during subjective sight testing, wherein the examiner repeatedly asks the patient to report which of two lens selections provides better vision until a final prescription determination is made. Patients would likely become upset if an apparently random series of prescription options was presented and the practitioner repeatedly inquired, "Is this one good enough for you?" Yet this is very much akin to the approach taken in AT assessments where consumers are exposed to few relevant device options. For example, an Arkansas study [6] found that almost half of blind and low visioned device recipients were unable to try out their devices before purchasing them. Although service professionals strongly encourage consumer involvement in the device selection process [7] [8], the specifics of this involvement are often vague and poorly documented. A significant exception is the approach advocated by Riemer-Reiss and Wacker [9], of Roger's [10] "diffusion of innovation theory." According to Rogers, there are five factors that affect the adoption or diffusion of any innovation: relative advantage, compatibility, complexity, trialability and observability. Of particular importance to assistive device selection and adoption are the concepts of trialability (the extent to which an innovation can be trialed and modified) and relative advantage (the extent to which an innovation is perceived to be better than others). Truly effective rehabilitation services can document the structure and support they provide that are necessary for consumers to make informed and rational decisions about their care (including the selection of appropriate devices). For consumers to have meaningful and constructive autonomy when selecting devices, there must be a methodical assessment protocol that goes beyond the exhortations given in the published literature in order to ensure that consumers are exposed to organized and systematic inter-device comparisons.

Device Abandonment

In spite of the considerable attention that goes into the AT assessment process, almost 30% of all prescribed devices are abandoned by their recipients within a relatively short period of time, often within four months of being purchased[9,11,12]. This is a post-dispensing reality that is easily ignored by device inventors, developers, vendors, and even service providers who often ignore this eventuality since most devices seem to be quite effective and well-received when they are dispensed to their intended users. Olkin [13] attributes the abandonment of assistive technology to "a complex interaction of many variables including characteristics of the user; utility, appropriateness, and match of the device to need(s); and availability of the assistive technology." Focus group research conducted by Batavia and Hammer[14] confirms that consumers will not successfully adopt and retain assistive devices unless they perceive the advantages of using the devices outweigh the burdens involved in their use. Consumers reported that the following four major problems with devices may result in their abandonment: (1) Inadequate performance of the device; (2) Failure to achieve suitably improved function with the device; (3) Difficulties with the device operation; (4) High costs for the device and its maintenance. Rogers and Holms [15] noted that problems arise when a device feels awkward, heavy, uncomfortable, or defective. Most of these device shortcomings can be anticipated and discussed with the patients before a device is prescribed.

No assistive devices are immune from abandonment, but some service providers boast significantly lower abandonment rates than others. Our experience has been that consumer satisfaction increases and the rate of abandonment decreases when considerable attention is paid to the device selection process. Others have similarly found that users are more likely to abandon their devices if their needs were not fully addressed during the selection process [16-21]. There appear to be many potential reasons why people discontinue using costly rehabilitation devices. Rarely are these devices abandoned because they no longer perform as well as they did at the time they were purchased. In a small number of cases, the user's needs or abilities may change unpredictably, making the device obsolete. The most common problem is that the device simply failed to meet all of the expectations of the purchaser. When this happens, people often blame it on the inappropriateness of the device. We contend that a more conspicuous culprit is the inappropriateness of the process that was used to select the device in the first place. The eventual disappointment often can be predicted before the device is purchased, but the critical indicators are missed or ignored during the assessment process.

Our Unique Service Environment

Our unique service environment was used to study

device-assisted rehabilitation strategies. The Centre for Sight Enhancement (CSE) is a large optometry-based clinical low vision service, research, and teaching facility at the University of Waterloo. With significant research and contract funding support, the CSE provides comprehensive low vision services that include high technology assessment and training services and an extensive electronic video device assessment service (for non-generic evaluation of portable, stationary, and head mounted video devices). Ours is the only Canadian low vision service to be externally accredited by the National Accreditation Council for Agencies Serving the Blind and Visually Handicapped. Our service activities are evaluated annually by two different government agencies from whom we receive funding, and by two professional Councils that oversee the education and research components of our activities. To survive under the constant scrutiny of such a varied mix of reviewers, we were compelled to develop a series of sound and defensible protocols for the assessment and training of all clients seen in our facility, regardless of their presentation or service/device needs[22]. We have a fairly extensive quality assurance program, which allows us to monitor self-reported client satisfaction and feedback. We have several ongoing research projects wherein post-service outcomes including functional status (VFQ-25) and psychosocial impact (PIADS) are sampled and analyzed extensively[1][23]. Our device infrastructure is supported in part by our longstanding involvement in the Assistive Devices Program (ADP), a government-sponsored program that provides funding support toward the purchase of any assistive devices that have been duly prescribed and authorized for Ontario residents with disabilities[24]. These include both high and low technology devices for disabilities in the categories of communication, respiration, mobility, ostomy, hearing, seating, prosthetics, orthotics, and vision. CSE researchers were asked to develop a series of sound and defensible protocols for the assessment and training of all low visioned clients being evaluated, regardless of their presentation or service/device needs [25]. The government's motivation was to safeguard against spending public monies for the purchase of unwarranted, ineffective, or excessive device technologies. This need for budgetary accountability is balanced by a desire to provide consumers with suitable autonomy in the device selection process. The resulting model recognizes the mutual compatibility of these two objectives. Most consumers recognize the detrimental impacts if unwarranted costs are incurred to purchase devices of limited utility, or if purchased devices are abandoned after a brief trial. It is also wasteful for consumers to lose time, energy, or hope, while working with an unsuitable device, when a better one is available.

Assessment Inventory Selection

To ensure that consumers obtain optimal assistive device assessment services in accordance with our CE approach, it is important for the service provider to actually have an appropriate inventory of devices available for assessment purposes. Assuming that such an array is available, it is equally important for the consumer to actually see and work with each potentially relevant device in the assessment inventory. Although low vision device topics dominate the low vision literature, [26] there has been little attention paid to the selection of the specific devices required for competent assessments or to the protocols for determining the most appropriate device for each service consumer, even in studies of intervention outcomes[27-33]. Regardless of the competencies of the assessor, the nature of the assessment will be significantly dependent on the precise array of devices available for the evaluation. Although researchers often differentiate service comprehensiveness by describing their multidiscipinarity,[34] the breadth of a service's device armamentarium provides another significant differentiation between secondary and tertiary levels of service [35]. The services provided by highly skilled and experienced service providers may be suboptimal when all of the requisite assets are unavailable. This demonstrates the reality that low vision assessments may be constrained by the various "assets" (personnel, infrastructure, and devices) available for these services.

A significant source of confusion for novice service providers working in the field of device-assisted vision rehabilitation is the large number of comparable devices that may be appropriate for each service consumer [36]. An expedient solution to this dilemma is to identify a calculated array of devices for assessment purposes such that the component devices are readily distinguishable from one another based on common differentiating characteristics such as application (for example, distance, intermediate, near, magnification, or light control), power (magnification level, fixed or variable), field of view, and form factor (hand, stand, spectacle-mounted, or head-borne; illuminated or non-illuminated)[35]. Mediated to some extent by clinical experience and manufacturer preferences, this is a common basis for devising low vision device "kits" for newer practitioners seeking to establish low vision assessment services in community practices. This ensures that a relevant and comprehensive array of devices is available for diverse patient encounters, while keeping the number of selection options to a manageable level. This may be considered to be an "asset-based" assessment protocol.When used in accordance with commonly accepted assessment protocols, these kits produce functionally effective and successful outcomes in approximately 90% of low vision cases encountered in primary care settings[37].

Depictions of comprehensive low vision assessment protocols typically use generic descriptives with exemplars to describe device inclusions in the assessment process. Generic inclusion criteria include mechanism (optical, non-optical, electro-optical, light control), application (distance, near or any distance), power (magnification range and inter-device intervals), form factor (spectacle-mounted, head-mounted, hand-held, stand, illuminated, or non-illuminated) and function (reading, mobility, seeing, and manipulation). Problems may arise when categories of potentially relevant devices are overlooked in the assessment kit. Unless they are evaluated by the consumers and service providers in accordance with the CE approach, their potential utility will remain uncertain. The emergence of a new category of video-based devices has been problematic [38]. As noted by Harper et al 1999,[39] the best way to confirm the relative utility of these new devices is to monitor their impact on quality of life in addition to more traditional measures of functional vision outcomes. This poses a service dilemma because "the cost and the time consuming nature of assessment and training prevents rehabilitation with these new systems from being encompassed" within existing low vision services.

Consumer Involvement in the Selection Process

Most clinicians are comfortable using quantitative performance measurements to establish an ordinal ranking for the presumed effectiveness of competing device interventions. For example, acuity resolution, reading speed, and reading endurance have been used to differentiate the potential utility of assistive devices for reading. Other non-performance factors are associated

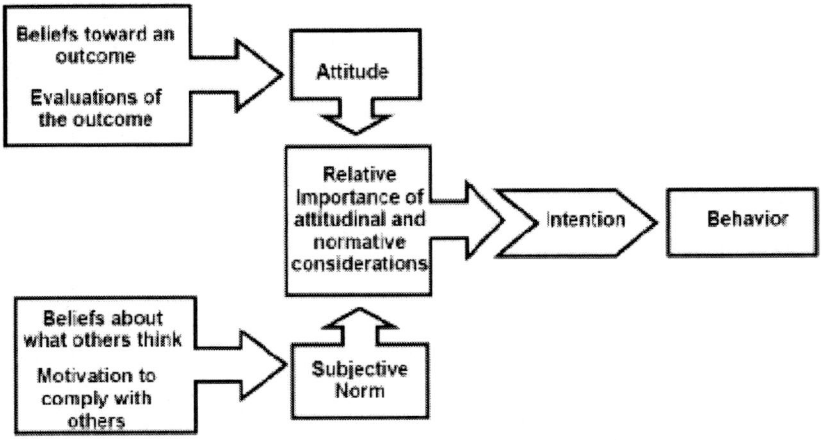

Figure 1. Reasoned Action Model (derived from Azjen & Fishbein, 1975)

with increased device usage and utility, including device cost, perceived aesthetics, operability, durability, versatility, efficiency, simplicity, comfort, ergonomics and safety[40-47]. Although these factors are highly individualistic and are almost impossible to integrate explicitly into a prescriptive protocol, they are incorporated implicitly when consumers are given an opportunity to make inter-device comparisons as with a CE protocol. Scherer et al [48] described a compelling framework for modeling the selection of assistive devices which acknowledges the primacy of the consumer in the process and recognizes how both subjective and objective needs impinge on the selection outcome.

It is possible to analyze some aspects of the assistive device selection process using standard consumer theory. The most enlightened purchase decisions are guided by the consumer's perception of what the consequences of the purchase will be, rather than how many features the product has. This is known as the "theory of reasoned action" (See Figure 1)[49] This theory also recognizes that the opinions of others (experts, significant others, and persons with similar disability) may have a significant impact on the consumer's selection[50].

The effort necessary for consumers to make complex purchase selections is significant. As a result, consumers frequently take shortcuts to reach a final decision. Rather than seeking the best device solution, they are willing to settle for a satisfactory solution. For example, they may decide to eliminate from consideration all devices that do not meet some criteria, such as cost or physical size. Although this helps to uncomplicate the final selection process, it may cause them to wrongly reject the "best" device. Another common approach is for consumers to identify what they believe to be the most important device feature, and base their decision solely on an inter-device comparison of this single feature. These are examples of what is called "satisficing"[51], because they often lead to satisfactory or acceptable purchase decisions, but rarely to ideal ones. Simon [52]contrasts the difference between optimizing as "looking for the sharpest needle in the haystack" and satisficing as looking for a needle in the haystack that is "sharp enough to sew with." Consumer advocates have suggested it is possible to help consumers by limiting their choices, or at least by organizing their choices in meaningful and constructive ways[48].

Decisions are usually made after aggregate values have been assigned to each available choice in accordance with some value-ordered heuristic[53]. Consumers are faced with a Goldilocks conundrum because they are unsure if any of the potentially available devices will be exactly right for their rehabilitation needs. Accordingly, they are willing to be somewhat flexible about their interpretation of "just right" and are inclined to stop testing when they find a solution that is "good enough."[54] Adding alternatives to a choice set has a complex influence on consumer judgments, which may become inconsistent with a simple cost-benefit trade-off model. It seems likely that assistive device "products" possess a variety of benefit and cost dimensions that may be contemplated in tandem when consumers evaluate the "relative advantage" of different devices. Problems arise when inter-device distinctions (such as magnification power) become so infinitesimal that participants are simply unable to decide among some of the device options available to them. The reverse condition may occur when inter-device distinctions (such as magnification power) become so coarse that participants sense that some potentially productive options are being under-explored. Another significant concern arises if the operant differentiating features for screening prospective devices fail to include any characteristics that are highly relevant for potential device users. Although many different devices may provide individual users with reasonable task proficiency, it seems reasonable to assume that among all of the devices that "work," only one or two will "work best." We sought to devise an assessment protocol that reliably identified the device(s) that worked best from among all of the devices that merely worked.

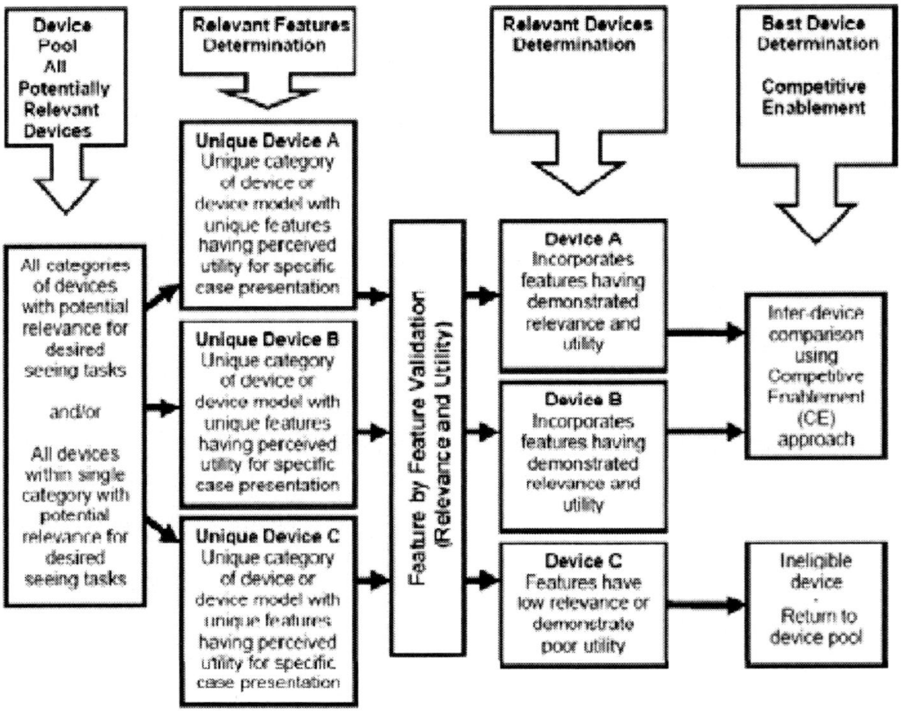

Figure 2 – Competitive Enablement – Device Selection Protocol
Final device selection may require cross-category or intra-category device comparisons using the CE approach. Cross category selection addresses different types of devices, such as hand magnifiers, spectacle magnifiers, stand magnifiers, and video magnifiers that all may be relevant and useful for specific reading activities. Some devices within each device category may exhibit "acceptable" utility for these intended activities. An inter-device comparison allows consumer to make a rational choice concerning which of these devices is the best one. Intra-category device selection deals with selecting from different types of devices within a single device category, such as video magnifiers being contemplated for specific reading activities. Some device models may be excluded because they have features (display enhancements, physical features, or ergonomics, for example) that are found to be "unacceptable" for these intended activities. An intra-device comparison of the remaining acceptable devices allows the consumer to make a rational choice concerning which model is best.

A systems development approach provides useful guidance for the selection of a specific device by a specific consumer. This process relies on a clear definition of the user, the user's goals, and the user's working environment. A CE approach ensures that consumers have the opportunity to factually compare the perceived utility of all devices that are potentially relevant for each component rehabilitation demand. In some instances, initial "relative advantage" perceptions may change when devices are trialled in habitual living environments. The person may experience changes in activity needs and expectations, in skills and abilities, or in the environmental context for the device[55]. When this eventuality is anticipated, devices may be loaned to the individual to verify their competitive utility in habitual settings. Alternatively, follow-up assessments may be conducted using the CE method to confirm the sustained utility of prescribed devices. The importance of structured follow-up assessments is well recognized in device-assisted rehabilitation[7].

Integrating New Device Technologies into the Selection Process

Assimilating new categories of devices or new features within existing device categories can be problematic for service providers who, in accordance with a CE approach, are anxious to include new and innovative products during the selection process. In the field of vision rehabilitation, for example, an ever-increasing number of video-based low vision products in the device marketplace poses an obvious dilemma for service providers and for service consumers. Portable video magnifiers introduce new form factors and enhancement options that are foreign to the traditional array of low vision devices available for assessments. In accordance with a CE philosophy these portable video devices should be evaluated alongside optical devices having competing enablement features (primarily magnification and form factor) to determine which device works best for the user. A number of adapted camera systems have emerged, which may be relevant for distance as well as near visualization tasks. Telescopes and telemicroscopes are relevant optical alternatives, against which video device performance can be evaluated. Some researchers have advocated demonstrating these new electro-optical devices only when appropriate for individual clients, but this assumes that service providers are able to make this determination and provides no mechanism for validating this capacity[56].

Figure 2 describes the process involved when evaluating the relative utility and relevance of competing devices from different device categories for each problematic seeing activity. A structured and rational approach is used to determine potentially eligible devices from each device category (such as telemicroscopes, hand magnifiers, stand magnifiers, spectacle magnifiers, and video magnifiers for reading). Some devices within each device category may exhibit "acceptable" utility for these desired activities. Service providers and consumers must be aware that the perceived relative utility of competing devices may change under different viewing conditions (such as dim light versus bright light; outdoors versus indoors; at near distances versus far distances). An inter-device comparison allows consumers to make a rational choice concerning which of these devices is the best one for each relevant condition. In some instances, multiple devices may be required to provide the best device disparate critical task conditions.

The selection process for high technology devices, such as closed circuit television (CCTV) systems, poses a different set of problems for service providers because the essential sight enhancement options (magnification and contrast enhancement) may be virtually identical for all of the competing products. However, this does not mean that they are interchangeably effective for individual users with different needs, expectations, and operating environments. Contemporary closed circuit (CCTV) systems offer an array of potentially relevant and differentiating options that cannot be explored realistically using a single CCTV assessment system. Further, it may be impossible to anticipate the relevance and effectiveness of these features based on observed performance using a generic CCTV device. Hence, inter-category device comparisons (comparing different stationary CCTV options) are required to demonstrate which CCTV device works best.

Figure 2 also describes the process involved when evaluating the relative utility and relevance of competing device models within a single device category. A structured and rational approach is used to determine potentially eligible devices within the device category (for example, different CCTV models with different display options, different ergonomic characteristics, different control options, different enhancement features, and different connectivity features). A single full-feature device can be used to investigate the utility of most display enhancement features, but inter-device comparisons are required to investigate ergonomic, control, and operational differences between competing models which may be critical for device utility. Some devices may be excluded because they have features that are irrelevant, ineffective, or unusable for the intended activities. An intra-device comparison of the remaining acceptable devices allows the consumer to make a rational choice concerning which model is best.

During the assessment, it is important to recognize the distinction between verified utility and probable utility. If someone wants to read a newspaper or a book, he should use each device under conditions that replicate or effectively simulate the circumstances of actual use, rather than simply reading a test card with different print samples. Some systems may work very well with clinical test samples, but fail miserably when used for reading the real material of interest under the actual conditions where it must be read. This approach also allows consumers to see how each device functions for prolonged reading tasks, if this is how they intend to use the system. Similarly, if the consumer wishes to use the system for reading foreign language material, household bills, or written correspondence, it is important to use real samples for evaluating each CCTV. The consumer should locate and use each control feature to allow him to compare any operating differences. This hands-on approach is particularly important for evaluating hand-operated camera systems or other out of line systems, where some consumers may experience considerable difficulty with tracking and alignment. The bottom line is to provide consumers with an opportunity to use each system in the way that they expect to use it after they have purchased it. In this way, a CE approach attempts to bridge the potential gap between efficacy and effectiveness.

In North America, many CCTV devices are purchased following isolated in-house demonstrations by device vendors. Notwithstanding the convenience and integrity of these services, these purchase decisions are constrained because they are usually made without due reference to other competing device options. A CE assessment protocol rigorously investigates the comparable utility of "lesser" devices (of lesser cost and sophistication) in the rehabilitation of explicit (identifiable and verifiable) disabilities for consumers, thus protecting consumers from obtaining sophisticated and expensive devices when other "lesser" devices might be equally or, even more appropriate. An exception to this may occur when changes are anticipated in the nature of a consumer's device needs, such as a foreseeable deterioration in the causal vision condition or pending changes in vision demands for various tasks. These concerns may be further exacerbated when consumers are locked into financial reimbursement programs (third party benefits) that preclude upgrading within a fairly lengthy time period (often at least five years). These circumstances may prompt consumers to opt for greater device functionality than is currently required.

The subjective incorporation of these qualitative determinants into the device selection process extends the concept of device-assisted rehabilitation beyond its traditional focus on functional status. Enhanced participation is now considered to be a key outcome for rehabilitation programs directed at assisting people with vision loss. With respect to service delivery, the concept of participation requires more attention to the broader issues of device-assisted persons functioning within their environments. The significance of this broader approach is well recognized in the occupational therapy assessment literature[57,58]. The concept of "environmental negotiability"[59] has been used to describe the extent to which a person can interact with his or her chosen environment. Translating this concept to vision rehabilitation, one might consider the "environment" as being the client's visual environment as opposed to the physical environment. Of particular relevance to persons with impaired vision are vision environments that are associated with performing various activities of importance where vision is a critical factor. Everyone has a unique "environment" which includes a large variety of potentially problematic activities, including those commonly associated with daily living (such as reading, writing, spotting, localizing, orienting, eating, grooming, self-care, and social interactions) as well as any activities that are more peculiar to individual consumer lifestyles (such as hobbies, vocations, and other interests). In general terms, the "environment" also includes any associated cultural, socio-economic, institutional, physical and social factors[60]. "Negotiability" describes the individual's self-rated capacity to interact effectively with his or her environment, and to perform all of the activities that he or she identifies as significant in his or her daily life. In other words, how well the person can do any of the things identified as being important in life. The concept of "environmental negotiability" is attractive because it reflects an individual's capacity to live life to its fullest, to participate in desired lifestyle with minimum limitations and restrictions. If this capacity is diminished by vision loss, it may be possible to be elevated or restored to some higher level using assistive devices. The relative impact of these devices is determined by the number of tasks that are affected, by their respective importance to the device user, and by the quality and extent of any improvements. This may explain why we have found that some of the devices that are best appreciated by consumers are those that have multiple uses, as opposed to those with one-dimensional applications. This realization surfaced in our work with head mounted video devices. Our follow-up interviews and confidential patient survey results revealed that people who obtained these devices in accordance with our CE assessment approach, rarely abandoned the selected devices (less than 5%), rarely abdicated their selected devices in favour of other competing devices (less than 2%), and usually reported increased device usefulness after becoming more familiar with its operation (more than 85%)[61].

Conclusion

Low vision devices should be selected in accordance with a Competitive Enablement (CE) approach. Service providers should offer consumers a suitable array of devices from which to choose, and it is important for consumers to base their purchase decisions on a competitive evaluation of the demonstrated utility and performance of these devices while using them to perform real seeing tasks. The true functional utility of competing devices can be evaluated by consumers when they are given an opportunity to use these devices for various seeing tasks that they identify to be both problematic and important. Consumers must also remain sensitive to other potential uses of the device for any additional activities that perhaps seem less worthy of mention when being interviewed by the service provider. With its cogent conceptual underpinning, this CE approach has the potential to fill an important gap in assistive device outcomes research between models for AT assessment.

References

[1] Strong G, Jutai JW, Bevers P, Hartley M, & Plotkin A. (2004) The psychosocial impact of closed-circuit television (CCTV) low vision aids. Visual Impairment Research, 5(3):179–190.

[2] Massof RW (2002) The Measurement of Vision Disability Optometry & Vision Science. 79(8):516-552.

[3] Agree EM (1999) The influence of personal care and assistive devices on the measurement of disability. Social Science & Medicine 48 (1999) 427-443.

[4] Jutai J, Hooper P, Strong J, Russell-Minda E, Cooper L, Hutnik C, Sheidow T, Tingey D. (2007). Vision rehabilitation evidence-based review: Module 1: Terminology, demography, and epidemiology of low vision. The University of Western Ontario, The Lawson Health Research Institute, and CNIB. Accessed (07/08/07) on-line at http://www.cnib.ca/en/about/publications/research/VREBR_Chap1_May2005.pdf

[5] Fuhrer MJ. (2001) Assistive technology outcomes research: Challenges met and yet unmet American Journal of Physical Medicine & Rehabilitation Volume 80(7), July 2001, pp 528-535.

[6] Parette H P, VanBiervliet A, & Holbrook MC. (1990). Technological needs of visually impaired and blind persons in Arkansas. Journal of Visual Impairment and Blindness, 84(10) 534-538.

[7] Cook AM, & Hussey SM. (2002). Assistive Technologies: Principles and Practice. 2nd edition St. Louis: Mosby.

[8] Scherer M.J. (2001). Matching consumers with appropriate assistive technologies. In D.A. Olson & F. DeRuyter (Eds), Clinician's Guide to Assistive Technology (pp. 3-13). St. Louis: Mosby.

[9] Riemer-Reiss ML & Wacker RR. (2000). Factors associated with assistive technology discontinuance among individuals with disabilities, Journal of Rehabilitation 66, 44-50.

[10] Rogers EM. (1995). Diffusion of innovations (4th ed.). New York: The Free Press.

[11] Phillips B & Zhao H. (1993). Predictors of assistive technology abandonment. Assistive Technology, 5, 36-45.

[12] Reimer-Reiss M. (2000). Assistive technology discontinuance. Paper presented at the CSUN Center on Disabilities - Technology and Persons with Disabilities Conference, (Denver) March 2000. Accessed (07/08/07) on-line at http://www.csun.edu/cod/conf/2000/proceedings/0003Reimer.htm

[13] Olkin R. (1999). What psychotherapists should know about disability. New York: The Guilford Press.

[14] Batavia AI & Hammer GS (1990). Toward the development of consumer-based criteria for the evaluation of assistive devices. J Rehab Res & Dev, 27, 425-436.

[15] Rogers JC & Holms MB (1992). Assistive technology device use in patients with rheumatic disease: A literature review. Amer J Occup Thera, 46, 120-127.

[16] Cook A (1982). Delivery of assistive devices through a client-oriented approach. In: Redden MR, Stern VW, editors. Technology for Independent Living II: Issues in Technology for Daily Living, Education and Employment. Washington: American Association for the Advancement of Science, pp. 29-31.

[17] Zola I (1982). Involving the consumer in the rehabilitation process: easier said than done. In: Redden MR, Stern VW, editors. Technology for Independent Living II: Issues in Technology for Daily Living, Education and Employment. Washington: American Association for the Advancement of Science, pp. 112-121.

[18] Carroll M & Phillips B (1993). Survey on assistive technology abandonment by new users (Cooperative Agreement No.H133E0016). Washington, DC: National Institute on Disability and Rehabilitation Research.

[19] Phillips B & Broadnax DD (1992). National survey on abandonment of technology (Cooperative Agreement No.H133E80016). Washington, DC: National Institute on Disability and Rehabilitation Research.

[20] Tewey BP, Barnicle K & Perr A (1994). The wrong stuff. Mainstream, 19(2), 19-23.

[21] Turner E, Barrett C, Cutshall A, Lacy BK, Keiningham J, & Webster MK (1995). The user's perspective of assistive technology. In: Flippo KF, Inge KJ, Barcus JM, editors. Assistive technology: A resource for school, work and community. Baltimore: Paul H. Brookes Publishing Co., pp. 283-290.

[22] Strong JG, Pace RJ, and Plotkin AD. (1988) Low vision services: a model for sequential intervention and rehabilitation. Canadian Journal of Public Health. 79 (S50 - S54).

[23] Strong G, Huber J, Taji R, Jutai J, Plotkin A, Ariizumi H. (2006)The relationship between measures of visual function and assistive device impact related to quality of life. Association for Research in Vision and Ophthalmology (ARVO), Fort Lauderdale, FL. May 4.

[24] Strong, JG (2001) Ontario Assistive Devices Program: A Managed Low Vision Care Network, in Vision Loss Rehabilitation: Service Delivery, Policy and Funding edited by Massof and Lidoff ed. AFB Press 2001

[25] Strong JG and Byard A. (1992) Protocols for the prescribing of non-generic closed circuit television (CCTV) systems for individuals with low vision. Invest. Ophthalmol. Vis. Sci. Suppl. 33. p.1417.

[26] Rosenbloom AA, Goodrich GL. (2000) Low vision research and development needs: differing perspectives, differing needs. In: Stuen C, Arditi A, Horowitz A, Lang MA, Rosenthal B, Seidman K, editors. Vision '99: Vision rehabilitation: assessment, intervention and outcomes. New York: Swets & Zeitlinger Publishers 19–22

[27] Leat SJ, Fryer A, Rumbey NJ. (1994) Outcome of low vision aid provision: The effectiveness of a low vision clinic. Optom Vision Sci. 71(3):199–206.

[28] Scott IU, Smiddy WE, Schiffman J, Feuer WJ, Pappas CJ. (1999). Quality of life of low-vision patients and the impact of low vision services. American Journal of Ophthalmology, 128(1):54–62.

[29] McCabe P, Nason F, Turco PD, Friedman D and Seddon JM. (2000) 'Evaluating the effectiveness of a vision rehabilitation intervention using an objective and subjective measure of functional performance', Ophthalmic Epidemiology, 7:4, 259 – 270 Accessed (07/08/07) on-line at http://dx.doi.org/10.1076/opep.7.4.259.4173

[30] Goodrich GL & Kirby J. (2001) A comparison of patient reading performance and preference: optical devices, handheld CCTV (Innoventions Magni-Cam), or stand-mounted CCTV (Optelec Clearview or TSI Genie). Optometry 72(8):519-528.

[31] Khan SA, Das T, Kumar SM, Nutheti R. Low vision rehabilitation in patients with age-related macular degeneration at a tertiary eye care centre in southern India. Clin Experiment Ophthalmol 2002;30(6):404-410.

[32] Reeves BC, Harper RA, Russell WB. (2004) Enhanced low vision rehabilitation for people with age related macular degeneration: a randomised controlled trial. Br J Ophthalmol 88(11):1443-1449.

[33] Landers A, Tapley J, Billington B, Almgill V, Mitchell-Baker A(1999) Cheaper can be better: Cutting costs and improving low vision aid service. British Journal of Visual Impairment, 17(3):111-115.

[34] Lovie-Kitchin JE, Whittaker SG. (1999) Prescribing near magnification for low vision patients. Clinical and Experimental Optometry 82(6):214-224.

[35] VISION 2020 Low Vision Group (2004) Standard List for Low Vision Services. Community Eye Health Vol 17 No. 49 Accessed (07/08/07) on-line at http://www.pubmedcentral.nih.gov/picrender.fcgi?artid=1705703&blobtype=pdf

[36] Wittich W, Strong JG, Renaud J and Southall K. (2007, in press) How to make low vision "sexy": A starting point for interdisciplinary student recruitment. RE:view (accepted for publication May 3, 2007).

[37] Elliott DB, Trukolo-Ilic M, Strong JG, Pace R, Plotkin A, and Bevers P. (1997) Demographic characteristics of the vision-disabled elderly. Investigative Ophthalmology and Visual Sciences (IOVS): 38(12) 2566-2575.

[38] Strong, G. (2004). New video-based assistive technologies for low vision. Journal of Vision, 4(11) Abstract 5, Page 5a. , Accessed (07/08/07) on-line at. http://journalofvision.org/4/11/5/

[39] Harper R, Culham L, and Dickinson C (1999) Head mounted video magnification devices for low vision rehabilitation: a comparison with existing technology Br. J. Ophthalmol. 83:495 - 500.

[40] Scherer MJ, & Lane JP. (1997). Assessing consumer profiles of 'ideal' assistive technologies in ten categories: An integration of quantitative and qualitative methods. Disability and Rehabilitation, 19(12), 528-535.

[41] Batavia AI, & Hammer GS. (1989). Consumer criteria for evaluating assistive devices: Implications for technology transfer. In J. J. Prosperin (Ed.), Proceedings of the 12 Annual Conference of Rehabilitation Engineering of North America (pp. 194-195). Washington, DC: RESNA Press.

[42] Reimer Reiss M and Wacker RR (1999) Assistive Technology Use and Abandonment among College Students with Disabilities International Electronic Journal

[43] Phillips B. (1993). Technology abandonment from the consumer point of view. National Rehabilitation Information Center Quarterly, 3, 1-10.

[44] Mallik K, & Elder G. (1993). Consumers who choose use... In M. Binion (Ed.), Proceedings of the RESNA 93 Annual Conference, Engineering the ADA (pp. 39-40). Washington, DC: RESNA Press.

[45] Brooks, N. A., & Hoyer, E. A. (1989). Consumer evaluation of assistive devices. In J. J. Presperin (Ed.), Proceedings of the 12th Annual Conference of the Rehabilitation Engineering Society of North America (pp. 358-359). Washington, DC: RESNA Press.

[46] Yaeda J, & Rubin SE. (1992). Job roles of assistive technology service providers in the United States. International Journal of Rehabilitation Research, 15, 277-287.

[47] Brienza D, Angelo J, & Henry K. (1995). Consumer participation in identifying research and development priorities for power wheelchair input devices and controllers. Assistive Technology, 7(1), 55-62.

[48] Scherer M, Jutai J, Fuhrer M, Demers L, DeRuyter F. (2007) A framework for modelling the selection of assistive technology devices (ATDs). Disability and Rehabilitation: Assistive Technology 2(1):1–8.

[49] Ajzen I. and Fishbein M.(1980), Understanding Attitudes and Predicting Social Behavior, Englewood Cliffs, NJ: Prentice-Hall,Inc.

[50] Ajzen I & Fishbein M. (1975) Belief, Attitude, Intention and Behavior: An Introduction to Theory and Research. Reading, Massachusetts: Addison-Wesley Publishing Co.

[51] Simon HA. (1987) Satisficing. In The New Palgrave: A Dictionary of Economics, Eatwell J, Millgate M, Newman P (eds.). Vol. 4: Stockton Press: New York; 243–245.

[52] Ibid. (page 244).

[53] Grundey D (2006) Delineating values, emotions and motives in consumer behaviour: an interdisciplinary approach // Transformations in business and economics 5(2): 21-46. Accessed (07/08/07) on-line at http://www.transformations.khf.vu.lt/10/articles/ge10.pdf

[54] Hulubei T, Freuder EC, and Wallace RJ (2003) The Goldilocks problem. Artificial Intelligence for Engineering Design, Analysis and Manufacturing AI EDAM (2003), 17: 3–11. Accessed (07/08/07) on-line at http://journals.cambridge.org/download.php?file=%2FAIE%2FAIE17_01%2FS0890060403171028a.pdf&code=062832327afc37f8d298f403f4d38dc7

[55] Arthanat S, Bauer SM., Lenker JA., Nochajski SM, and Wu YWB. (2007) Conceptualization and measurement of assistive technology usability. Disability and Rehabilitation: Assistive Technology. 2(4):235–248.

[56] Culham LE, Chabra A, Rubin GS (2004)Clinical performance of electronic, head-mounted, low-vision devices Ophthalmic and Physiological Optics 24(4):281-290.

[57] Christiansen, C. & Baum, C. (1997) Person-environment occupational performance: an occupation-based framework for practice. In: Occupational Therapy: Enabling Function and Well Being, Third Edition (eds C. H. Christiansen & C. M. Baum), pp. 46–79. Slack Incorporated, Thorofare, NJ, USA.

[58] Rousseau J, Potvin L, Dutil E, Falta P. (2001) Occupational Therapy In Health Care 14(3/4) 93-104.

[59] Norris-Baker C, & Willems EP. (1979). Environmental negotiability as a direct measurement of behavior-environment relationships: Some implications for theory and practice. In A. D. Seidel, & S. Danford (Eds.), Environmental design: Research, theory and application (pp. 209-214). Washington, D. C.: Environmental Design Research Association.

[60] Law M, Cooper B, Strong S, Stewart D, Rigby P, & Letts L. (1996). The person–environment–occupation model: A transactive approach to occupational performance. Canadian Journal of Occupational Therapy, 63, 9– 23.

[61] Strong JG. (1996) The Low Vision Enhancement System (LVES): Understanding a new generation of video devices. CNIB "Sharing the Vision" Conference, Lake Joseph, Ontario (June 10, 1996).

[62] Fuhrer MJ, Jutai JW, Scherer MJ & DeRuyter F. (2003). A framework for the conceptual modelling of assistive technology device outcomes. Disability and Rehabilitation. 25(22):1243-1251.

[63] Jutai JW, Fuhrer MJ, Demers L, Scherer MJ, DeRuyter F. (2005) Toward a taxonomy of assistive technology device outcomes. American Journal of Physical Medicine & Rehabilitation 84(4):294 – 302.

Aging, Disability and Independence
W.C. Mann (Ed.)
IOS Press, 2008

doi:10.3233/978-1-58603-902-8-197

New Approach to Ultrasonic Urine Sensor

Hiroyuki KODAMA[a,1], Hisashi YOSHIMURA[b], Kejin HUANG[c], Jing YU[a], Naoki ICHIKAWA[a], Ryutaro MAEDA[a], Yoshihiko NAGATA[a], Mitsuo WADA[d]
[a] Advanced Manufacturing Research Institute, Institute of Advanced Industrial Science and Technology, Tsukuba 305-8564, Japan
[b] Takeshiba Electric Co., Ltd., Kanagawa 3371-32, Japan
[c] Beijing University of Chemical Technology, Beijing 10039, People's Republic of China
[d] Hokkaido University, Sapporo 060-0808, Japan

Abstract. An ultrasonic urine sensor was developed to improve the quality of life for older people with urinary incontinence. The sensor was first designed for medical use and is now used in the clinical guideline of the Japanese Urological Association. Improvements were undertaken to make the sensor easy to use. The new approach is described in this paper.

Keywords. Urinary incontinence, bladder, urine, posture sensor

Introduction

In Japan, there are now about 27 million people over age 65, approximately one fifth of the population. It is estimated that 4.4 million require care, and this number will continue to increase. Urinary incontinence is a common problem. Technology to address this problem is an important area.

In a medical examination, consideration of urine residual is an important aspect for diagnosing urine voiding capability. Assisted urine voiding is an important aspect of nursing care. Unfortunately, detemining urine residual for diagnosis of internal pressure is highly painful and invasive, and suffering also occurs as a result of forced adaptation to the use of diapers. The ultrasonic urine sensor, capable of easily detecting bladder volume from outside the human body, will be very beneficial for patients.

The ultrasonic urine sensor is now sold to hospitals and is described in the clinical guidelines of the Japanese Urological Association. It is an accepted instrument for measuring urine residual. Moreover, since the device can also be used to reflect the dynamics of urine storage and voiding, it can be helpful in determining the urine voiding ability of a patient.

An area of future research is to further evolve the ultrasonic urine sensor into an apparatus that can be used with ease by not only medical specialists such as doctors, nurses and caregivers, but also by patients and their family members. To achieve this, significant improvements have been made including modification of the principle of measurements itself.

Method

To evaluate the measurement index of the ultrasonic urine sensor, an MRI test was carried out. Consent was first obtained from the study participants. Next, the shape changes of the bladder were gradually enlarged, and measured by a MRI made by SIEMENS Inc. During the intervals of MRI testing, measurement with the ultrasonic urine sensor was also conducted. For augmenting the urine voiding, the persons tested were asked to drink water.

To reduce the zigzag nature of the measurements caused by the use of ultrasound, various mathematical processing methods were tried. Methods to improve the measurement accuracy were studied in terms of the corresponding relationship between the

Table 1. Results of MRI measurement

subject	age	body type	voided volume	MRI calculation	residual urine
1F	34	plump	147ml 850ml	157ml 799ml	22ml
2F	38	slender	187ml 251ml 123ml	227ml 284ml 153ml	46ml
3M	31	standard	86ml 346ml	109ml 382ml	31ml
4F	30	standard	110ml 459ml	120ml 529ml	17ml
5F	27	slender	291ml 570ml	158ml 504ml	57ml
6F	35	standard	136ml 284ml	134ml 281ml	none
7M	49	standard	69ml 483ml	64ml 472ml	none
8F	35	slender	244ml 450ml	147ml 323ml	none
9F	35	standard	132ml 488ml	102ml 581ml	51ml
10M	34	stout	114ml 244ml	133ml 236ml	23ml

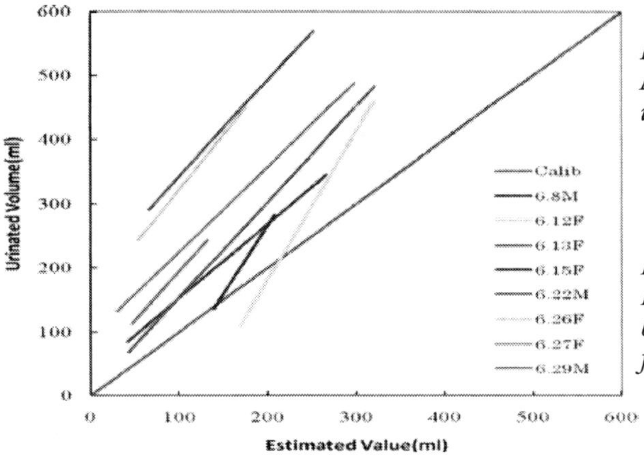

Figure 1. (left) Measurements by ultrasonic sensor

Figure 2. (below) Different shapes of full bladder and common features of bladder filling

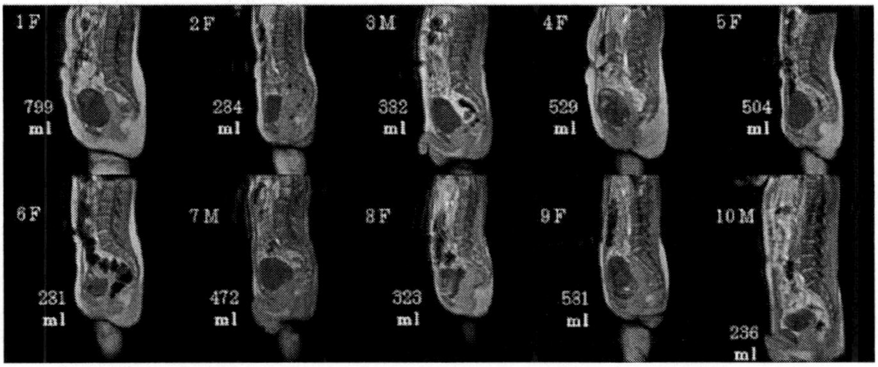

amount of urine in the bladder and the output of the ultrasonic urine sensor in case of urine voiding.

Owing to the shape change of the bladder in the human body, it is necessary to maintain a good condition for the ultrasound to transfer between the probe and the patient. However, it is not easy to realize this because of the movement of human body caused by breathing and other activities, hence intensifying the zigzag nature of the measurements. Moreover, the position and

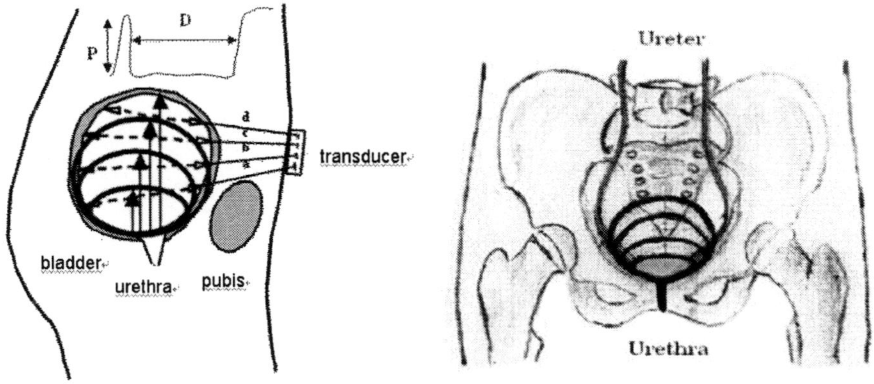

Figure 3. Upward shape change from the bottom of the bladder

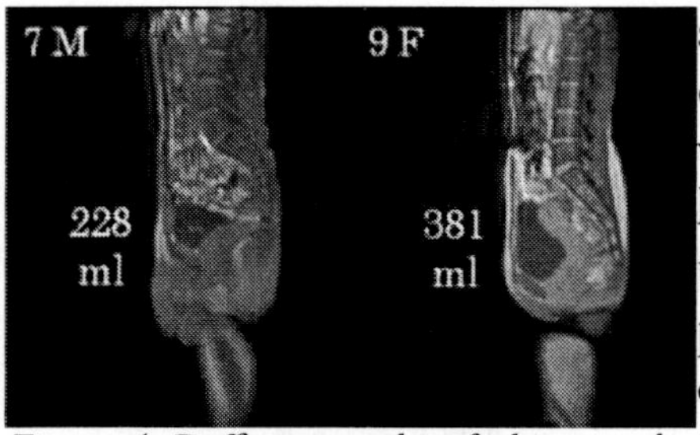

Figure 4. Different angles of ultrasound to the back wall of the bladder

shape of the bladder is different due to influences of the intestine when the person is standing or lying. Even in a lying posture, the relative location of the probe and the bladder can be different depending on whether the person is on one's back or side. The supine posture was used for the ultrasonic urine sensor. With the help of the posture sensor, measurement accuracy can be maintained in the supine posture even when the person is performing activities of daily life.

Results and Discussions

Ten participants (three men and 7 women) in good health were recruited to measure bladder variation. In Table 1 the

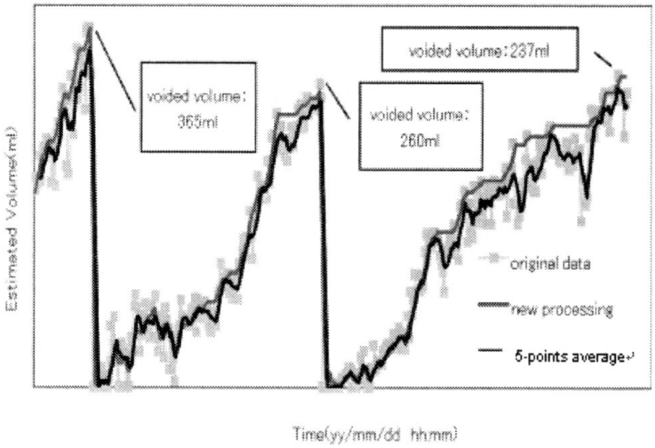

Figure 5. Processing to reduce the zigzag nature of the measurements

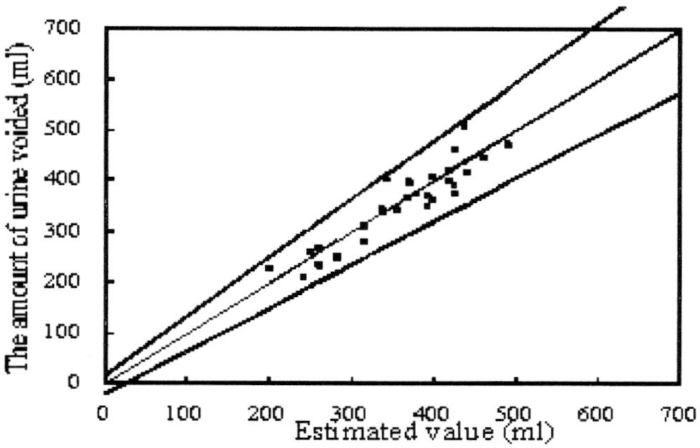

Figure 6. Analysis of 29 measurements in 9 days experiment by the least squares method

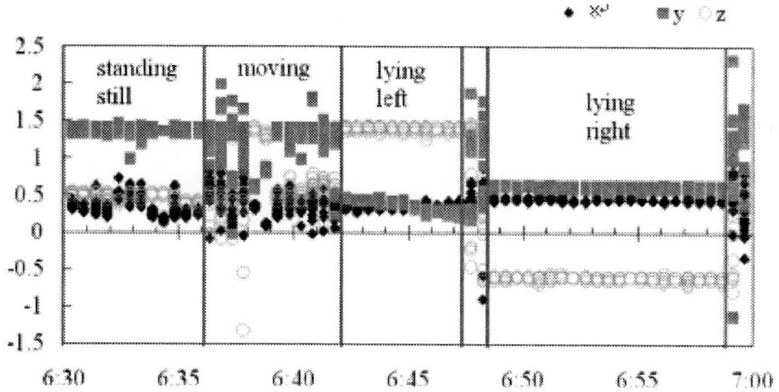

Figure 7. Processing to reduce the zigzag nature of the measurements

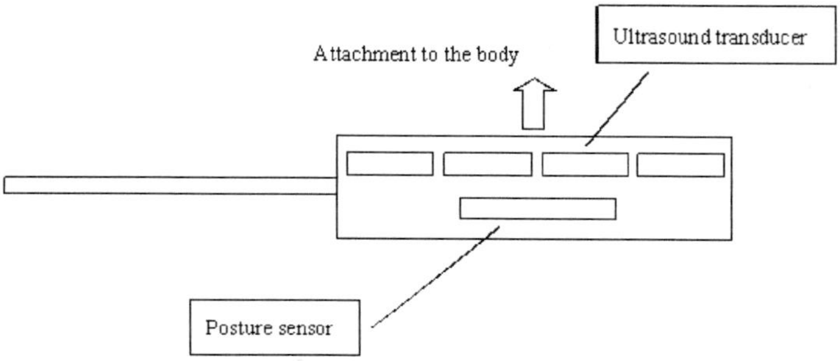

Figure 8. Analysis of 29 measurements in 9 days experiment by the least squares method

detailed outcomes are tabulated. Caused by the augment of the bladder, the increasing tendency of the measurements by the ultrasonic urine sensor was identified as is shown clearly in Figure 1. With regard to accuracy, good agreement was obtained (c.f., the difference between the measurements and Calib line), however, further improvement is possible.

Different shapes of full bladder and common features of bladder filling the position of the probe were taken into consideration. In Figure 2, the shape of the bladder was photographed with MRI. Although the patterns differed, common features were extracted, i.e., the bottom of the bladder can be seen as the base and the primary augment occurs toward the top. As shown in Figure 3, the right and left ureter from the kidney connect the bladder and open to the urethra. It is readily understood that the right and left ureter and the opening to the urethra approximate the shape of a right triangle. The wall of the bladder within this area is sharply different from that of the other part, which accounts for the difference in the echoes obtained from them. The measurement index used in the current ultrasonic urine sensor has not taken account of the difference. As shown in Figure 4, if different angles are considered in sending the ultrasound signal from each element to the back wall of the bladder, the currently employed measurement index, can still be used in the formulation to improve the accuracy of measurement. The weighting factor "wi" plays an important role.

Figure 5 shows the result of reducing the zigzag nature of the measurements. The sensitivity of the measurements was reduced considerably with a 5-point moving average algorithm. With this new processing method, the ultrasonic urine sensor can now predict the augment of the bladder with reasonable accuracy and with no occasional decrease of the outputs, except in urine voiding.

In Figure 6, the experimental results are illustrated for the same person for 29 measurements over the 9 day experiment. With the use of the formulation, V=C0*PD+C1, where its parameters are obtained by the least squares method, thre is improvement of the corresponding relationship between the outputs of ultrasonic urine sensor and the amount of urine voided. With the inclusion of the parameters, C0 and C1, the optimal value of the bladder volume can be determined.

In Figure 7, the experimental results of a three-dimensional accelerometric sensor fixed on an animal are displayed. The value on the x, y and z axis indicates the position variations of the animal when in standing, and in lying on the left and right side, respectively. With the application of this information, reliable measurements can be obtained by the ultrasonic urine sensor not only when the patient lies on his back, but also when he is active, provided that the relative location between the probe and the bladder is maintained.

Based on this promising accelerometric sensor data, a new composition of ultrasound transducers and a posture sensor produced by accelerometric sensor is illustrated in Figure 8.

Conclusions

The effectiveness of the ultrasonic urine sensor has been generally confirmed by a number of applications, ranging from use as an instrument for the detection of urine residuals to training in nursing departments of several universities. The ultrasonic urine sensor has been improved by alleviating the zigzag nature of its measurements through time series analysis, improving the measurement index, and using the position sensor.

References

[1] Kodama, H., Yu, J., Iwatsubo, E., Kuchinomachi, Y., Yoshimura, H., Kuchitsu, N.K. An Ultrasonic Urine Sensor for Aged People On Proceedings of the International Conference on Aging & Disability (ICADI). University of Florida (2006)

[2] Kodama, H., Huang, K., Yu, J., Kuchinomachi, Y., Yoshimura, H., Wada, M. Development of a New Ultrasonic Urine Sensor for Bladder Measurement Trans. of the Society of Instrument and Control Engineers, Vol.43, No.3, pp.156-165 (2007)

[3] Kodama, H., Huang, K., Yu, J., Nagata, Y., Yoshimura, H. An Ultrasonic Urine Sensor for Caregiving On Proceedings of the Festival of International Conferences on Caregiving, Disability, Aging and Technology (FICCDAT). Toronto, Canada (2007)

Aging, Disability and Independence
W.C. Mann (Ed.)
IOS Press, 2008

doi:10.3233/978-1-58603-902-8-205

Closed-Captions for Viewers with Low Vision Caption Speed and New Tools

Shigeki Inoue (Hakuhodo),
Yasushi Nakano (Keio University)
Tetsuya Arai (Keio University), Nobuyuki Nagai (Miyagi University of Education) Kensuke Ooshima (Tokyo Metropolitan University)
Yuriko Yamamoto (Graphic Designer), Nicole Schepker (Adaptive Environments)

Abstract: In an era in which the world population of individuals aged 65 and older constitutes nearly 500 million people, the accessible design of information is increasingly important. Closed-captioning, originally designed to make televised information accessible to deaf and hearing-impaired individuals, now benefits millions of people with a wide range of abilities. The United States, which has legislated captioned television for over thirty years, can be considered a world leader in the practice from which many countries, including Japan, may learn. Yet even in the U.S. there is no effective style of captioning for elders and people with low-vision. The captioning of short clips, such as TV commercials and short video, is especially lacking.

In our research we are establishing a methodology for appropriate captions for people with low vision, based on the Universal Design process pertaining to TV commercials. In Experiment 1 we examined the ways participants' visual behaviors were affected when their visual acuity was artificially reduced while viewing closed-captions, and the effects of reduced visual acuity on contents comprehension. In Experiment 2 we examined the participants' eye movement as they watched Japanese closed-captions at various speeds with no sound.

We realized that 1) participants' tended not to look at the captions when their visual acuity was reduced making it more difficult to read, 2) for participants with visual acuity lower than 0.25, captions were unreadable, 3) participants were affected by the caption speed when they had diminished visual acuity, and thus, they could not see the caption, and 4) eye movement is a valid index in researching people's viewing and comprehension of film clips. The results also indicate that closed-captions are currently unsuitable for viewers with lowered visual acuity, even for those viewers with slightly reduced visual acuity.

We now know that we must develop closed-captions that consider viewers with low-vision. We also know that total fixation time on captions calculated from eye movement is an especially valuable tool for researching the visual behaviors of viewers. This technology will not only aid the captioning process, but will also make the growing areas of new and online media accessible to millions of people.

U.S. Caption Viewing Audience by Category

- **28 Million Deaf and hard of hearing people**
- **47 Million People for whom English is a second language**
- **35 Million Illiterate adults improving their reading skills**
- **17 Million Children learning to read**
- **5.8 Million Remedial Readers**
- **Millions of others who watch television in bars, restaurants, airports, health & fitness clubs and hospitals.**

—NCI

Figure 1. U.S. Caption Viewing Audience by Category

Introduction

In an age of worldwide unprecedented growth in the elderly population, there is also an increasing incidence in hearing and vision loss and other age-related disabilities. It is imperative that we seek to extend accessibility in all areas of life. According to the U.S. Census Bureau, the world population of individuals aged 65 and older exceeded 495 million in mid-year 2007; as the population pyramid continues to invert, approriate accessible design, including application of the principals of universal design, must be considered to meet the needs of this population.

Television viewing is a routine activity for most people. Since the development of closed-captioning in the late twentieth century deaf and hearing-impaired individuals have gained access to televised information in many countries. The practice, however, should not only be expanded to reach an even broader range of people, but should be improved for the benefit of individuals with visual impairments that may hinder their ability to read and enjoy captions. In the U.S. alone there are approximately 8.7 million people with visual impairments [1].

An effective way to caption for elders and people with low-vision has not been developed adequately, nor has a standard style been established. The captioning of short clips, such as TV commercials and short video, is especially lacking.

The purpose of our research is to establish a methodology for providing appropriate captions for people with low vision based on the principals of universal design applied to TV commercials. In the first experiment, we examined the participants' visual behaviors when they saw common closed-captions on screen. In the second experiment we focused on examining the participants'

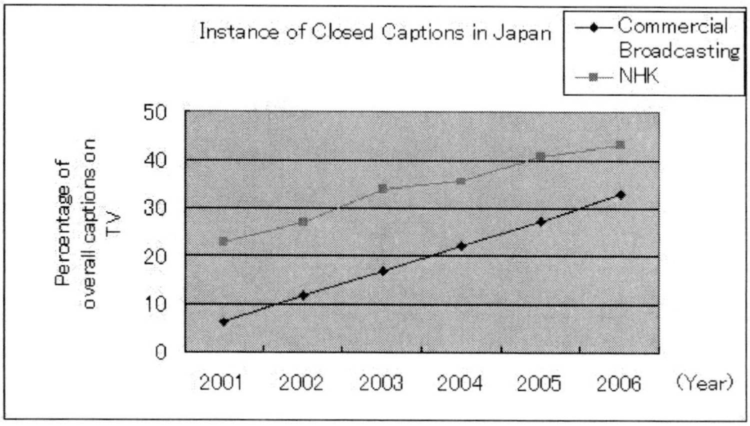

Figure 2. Instance of Closed Captions in Japan

visual acuity as they viewed the closed-captions at various speeds. This experiment used a TV commercial and the appropriate index from the first experiment.

To illustrate how captioning may be expanded globally, we have provided a brief review of the major events that led to the U.S. expansive caption viewing audience and the improvements being made to the captioning process in Japan.

Closed-Captioning in the United States and Japan

Closed captioning was developed to address the needs of the deaf. Today, there are millions of people accessing closed captioning in the U.S. in addition to the 28 million Americans who consider themselves deaf or hearing-impaired. The National Captioning Institute (NCI) asserts that the U.S. caption viewing audience consists of over 100 million people, or one third of U.S. residents (see Figure 1)[3].

U.S. captioning began in 1972 with PBS's cooking show The French Chef and The Captioned ABC Evening News in 1973. Seventeen years later, closed-captioning experienced two revolutionary federal laws. The first, the Television Decoder Circuitry Act of 1990, required all new television sets 13 inches or larger manufactured for sale in the U.S. to contain a caption-decoder chip. The second was the Americans with Disabilities Act, which required any public service announcements (PSA) funded solely or partially by the U.S. Federal government to include closed-captioning.

In 1996 the Telecommunications Act was passed, establishing the implementation of 100% captioning of new (aired 1998 and later) non-exempt English and Spanish language programming by 2006 and 2010, respectively, and 75% captioning of "old" (aired prior to 1998) non-exempt English and Spanish programming by 2008 and 2012, respectively. Exemptions to these rules can be either self-implementing or based on undue burden (FCC, 2007). Since 2000, the FCC has recommended that broadcasters who provide emergency information do so in an accessible format for deaf and hearing-impaired individuals as part of the Telecommunications Act.

In 1998 Section 508 of the Rehabilitation Act was passed, requiring all Federal departments and agencies to provide both employees and members of the general public with disabilities access to information comparable to that which individuals without disabilities receive. Section 508 refers to the development, procurement, maintenance and use of Federal electronic and information technology [6].

In Japan, closed-captioning has been used for over thirty

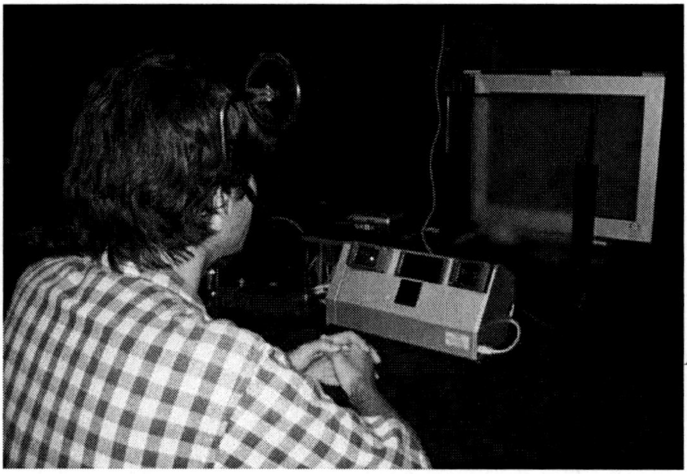

Figure 3

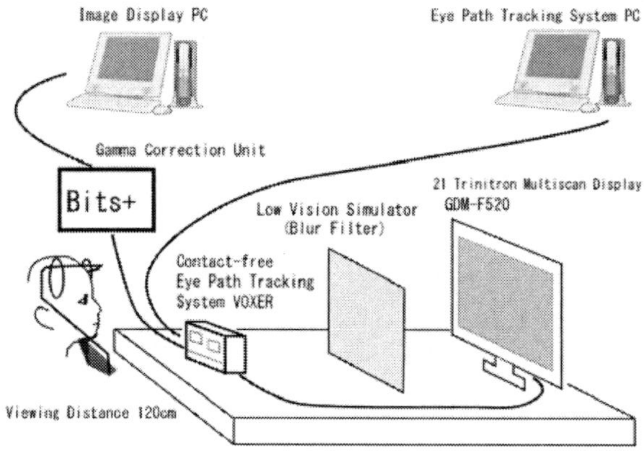

Figure 4

years, yet the amount of captioning remains below 50%, despite increases among both public and private broadcasters over the past five years. The Ministry of International Affairs and Communication recommended that major Japanese broadcasters adopt closed-captioning for all programs in 1997. In 2007, the Ministry reported 43.1% captioning on public broadcasting network NHK and a 32.9% captioning rate across the five major commercial broadcasting networks (Figure 2).

Although the U.S. is the captioning leader, there are still no captioning regulations for TV commercials 5 minutes in length or less, non-Federal websites, and online media. In Japan, there are no captioning regulations at all, only recommendations. Based on the following observations, however, we believe captioning will not only have the opportunity to increase in Japan and the U.S., but across the world.

Experiment 1

The purpose of experiment one was to analyze participants' visual behavior when viewing Japanese closed-captions with artificially reduced visual acuity. It is difficult for people with low vision to see and read closed-captions. When people view films in languages that are not their own, they do not gain information from the words spoken. Closed-captions play an important role for these films. In this experiment, we examined how participants' visual behaviors were affected when their visual acuity was artificially reduced while viewing a screen with closed-captions. We then analyzed the results by using their eye movement and contents comprehension as an index.

Methods

We examined the participants' eye movement while they viewed a film by using the remote eye movement-tracking device (Figure 1). The measurement device was composed of three mechanical units: (a) the image presentation device to show the image with Gamma correction, (b) the measurement device (VOXER, nac Image Technology Inc.) to record the participants' eye movements, and (c) the blur filter to simulate various low resolution conditions (Figures 3 & 4).

(a) Image Presentation Device: CRS (Cambridge Research Systems Ltd.) BITS++ and our self-made Gamma correction software, simulating TV color on a PC screen, were used to show the film with closed-captions on a Sony flat screen 21 trinitron multiscan display GDM-F520. The viewing distance between the users and the screen was 120cm (47.2 in). CRS COLOR CAL was used to measure light for the Gamma correction. CANVASs Co., Ltd. SST G1 was used to play the film, which was shown in full-screen.

(b) Eye Tracking System: As the remote eye tracking system, nac EMR-AT VOXER (sampling frequency of 60 Hz), was used to record the participants' fixation. The participants were provided with a chinrest and headrest to stabilize their head to obtain accurate examination records.

(c) Low Vision Simulator/ Blur Filter: The low vision simulator (Nakano et al, 2006) – blur filter – was used to artificially

Figure 5

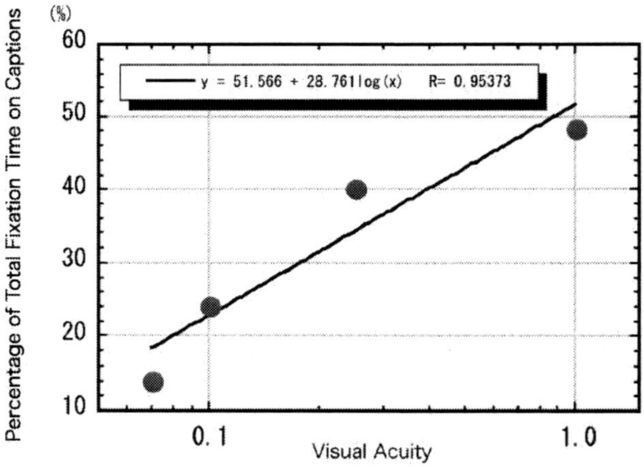

Figure 6

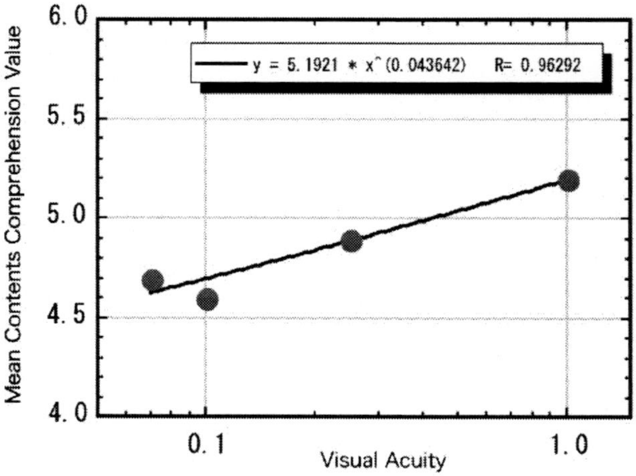

create various low-vision conditions by changing the distance between the screen and the filter. The simulated visual acuities were (average) 1.0, 0.25, 0.1, and 0.07 vision at filter distances of: no filter, 10 cm (3.9 in), 30 cm (11.8 in), and 50 cm (19.7 in), respectively.

We created 8 one-minute film clips with Japanese closed-captions and no sound from the SF entertainment movie 'Short Circuit.' Each film was played after a 5-second count down image was shown on screen. We had 4 simulated visual acuity conditions (filter distances: no filter, 10 cm, 30 cm, and 50 cm [1.0, 0.25, 0.1, 0.07]), and we experimented twice with each condition. Thus, we had a total of 8 trials. After participants viewed the film with Japanese closed-captions and no sound, we asked them several questions regarding the film. Participants included 5 Japanese adults (2 male and 3 female) with no visual impairments.

Results

Eye Movement: We calculated the percentage of the participants' fixation on the captions from their eye tracking data and called it the percentage of total fixation time on captions. It was calculated as "(the duration users' eyes were fixed on closed-captions ÷ the duration closed-captions were shown) × 100." The mean percentage of fixation on captions is indicated by visual acuity (Figure 5). The data affirms that as visual acuity was reduced, the percentage of caption viewing also decreased.

Contents Comprehension:

We examined the accuracy of the participants' answers regarding film contents. We asked 3 new participants to examine the answers by comparing them to the actual film clips, and to create 10-point rating scale. We then calculated the mean values from the results, and referred to them as the mean contents comprehension value. The mean value of all participants' contents comprehension is indicated by visual acuity in Figure 6. The results of Figures 5 and 6 indicate similar tendencies; however, the difference is more apparent in the percentage of total fixation time on captions.

Discussion

We discovered that with lowered visual acuity the percentages

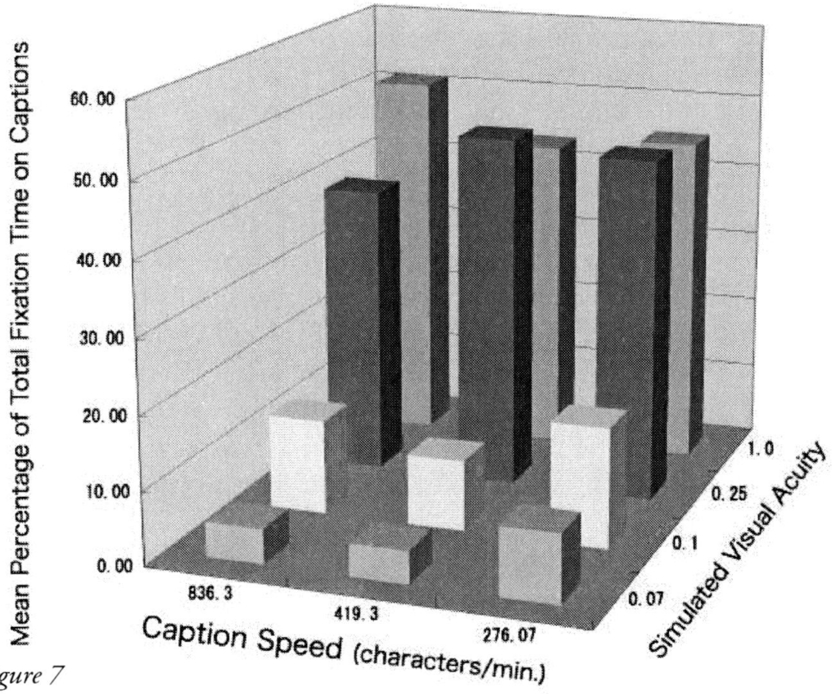

Figure 7

declined for both (total) fixation time of captions and contents comprehension. For participants with visual acuity lower than 0.25, the closed-captions were almost unreadable. These results indicate that the closed-captions currently used in Japan are unsuitable for viewers with lowered visual acuity, even for those viewers with slightly reduced visual acuity. We now know that we must develop closed-captions that consider the needs of low-vision viewers.

The results of the total fixation time on captions and contents comprehension tests revealed similar tendencies; however, the percent differences among visual acuities were narrower in contents comprehension. Users gathered contents information through the images rather than the captions.

Thus, the results and data from both experiments are considered a usable index for measuring the effectiveness of captions, though, the eye tracking results will be a more valuable index when evaluating how viewers see and gather information from both images and captions.

Experiment 2

Experiment two explored the effects of reduced visual acuity and caption speed on participants' visual behaviors. It was clear from the results of Experiment 1 that the participants' tendency was not to look at the captions when their visual acuity declined making it more difficult to read the captions. In Experiment 2 we examined how this visual behavior toward captions was affected by the display speed.

Methods

We followed the same protocol, used the same equipment, and the same 5 participants as in Experiment 1: we displayed the film on a screen with Japanese closed-captions and no sound, and examined the participants' eye movement while they watched the film by using the remote eye tracking system. To establish a 'real' TV commercial viewing condition, we used a film developed to improve children's visual recognition and added dummy captions. An excerpt from a middle school Japanese textbook was used for captioning. The length of the film was 20 seconds. We had 4 visual acuity conditions (1.0, 0.25, 0.1, 0.07), and 3 caption display speeds (characters per minute: 267.1 characters/min, 419.3 characters/min, and 836.3 characters/min). We experimented twice with each condition (4 visual conditions × 3 caption display speeds × 2 = 24 experiments). Thus, we had a total of 24 trials. The Participants were asked to view a 20-second film and to answer questions regarding the film's contents.

Results

We calculated the percentage of participants' fixation on captions from their eye movement data and called it the percentage of total fixation time on captions. It was calculated using the same equation as in Experiment 1. For each visual acuity condition and caption speed we indicated the mean percentage of total fixation time on captions (Figure 7). Overall, we recognized that participants were affected by the caption speed when they had a lowered visual acuity condition, and thus, they did not see the caption. We also realized that each visual acuity condition had a peak percentage of total fixation time on captions at different caption speeds: 1.0 visual acuity, the fastest caption speed; 0.25 visual acuity, the second fastest caption speed; 0.1 and 0.07 visual acuity, the slowest caption speed.

Discussion

Similar to Experiment 1, we discovered that the lower the visual acuity, the lower the percentage of total fixation time on captions. This experiment also revealed that the lower the visual acuity, the more participants were affected by the caption speed.

At least within the scope of this experiment, it was clear that for participants with normal visual acuity the fastest caption speed did not have much effect, and that participants did not have difficulty reading the captions or comprehending the contents. However, the caption speed had a significant effect on the participants with lowered visual acuity, and it acted as an obstacle to their reading and comprehension.

Conclusion

As stated, it is important to have captions on TV programs, movies, websites, and TV commercials in order to communicate with and inform the greatest number of people. In this study, we discovered that eye movement was one of the valid indexes in researching people's viewing and comprehension of the film clips. When viewers need to see both images and captions, such as with TV commercials, the percentage of total fixation time on captions calculated from eye movement is an especially valuable tool for researching viewers' visual behaviors.

Acknowledgement

We would like to extend special thanks to Larry Goldberg, Director of Media Access at WGBH, for his generous guidance throughout the writing process.

References

[1] Blindness Statistics. 2007. American Foundation for the Blind. 25 Oct. 2007 <http://www.afb.org/Section.asp?SectionID=15#num>

[2] Closed Captioning: FCC Consumer Facts. 29 Aug. 2007. Federal Communications Commission. 24 Oct. 2007 <http://www.fcc.gov/cgb/consumerfacts/closedcaption.html>

[3] Corporate Sponsorship. NCI The Global Captioning Leader. 11 July 2007. <http://www.ncicap.org/corpspon.asp>

[4] Ministry of International Affairs and Communication Japan. "ICT Policy." 2007

[5] Nakano, Y., Arai, T., Nagai, N., Nunokawa, K., Kusano, T., Maebashi, N., (2006). Developing an Evaluation System for Legibility as a Universal Design Tool: Advantages of a low vision simulator utilizing a wide view ground glass filter, The 2nd International Conference for Universal Design, in Kyoto 2006, P-022.

[6] Robson, Gary D. The Closed Captioning Handbook. Burlington, MA: Focal Press, 2004 Table 094. Midyear Population, by Age and Sex. U.S. Census Bureau, International Data Base, 16 Oct. 2007, http://www.census.gov/cgi-bin/ipc/idbagg

W.C. Mann (Ed.)
IOS Press, 2008

Author Index